A. Jay Stevens

The Star Quizzer on Pharmacy, Chemistry and Materia Medica

A. Jay Stevens

The Star Quizzer on Pharmacy, Chemistry and Materia Medica

ISBN/EAN: 9783742816856

Manufactured in Europe, USA, Canada, Australia, Japa

Cover: Foto ©Lupo / pixelio.de

Manufactured and distributed by brebook publishing software
(www.brebook.com)

A. Jay Stevens

The Star Quizzer on Pharmacy, Chemistry and Materia Medica

STUDENT SERIES.

THE STAR QUIZZER

ON

PHARMACY, CHEMISTRY AND MATERIA MEDICA

DESIGNED FOR

THE USE OF PHARMACEUTICAL STUDENTS PREPAR-
ING THEMSELVES FOR ADVANCED STANDING IN
COLLEGES OF PHARMACY AND FOR PREPARING
TO PASS THE STATE PHARMACEUTICAL EX-
AMINATIONS OF THE VARIOUS STATES.

BY

A. JAY STEVENS, Ph. G.
REGISTERED PHARMACIST.

AND

CHAS. W. MALLORY, Ph. G.
REGISTERED PHARMACIST.

PRICE, $1.25, POSTPAID.

PUBLISHED BY
STEVENS & MALLORY
ADA, OHIO.

Preface.

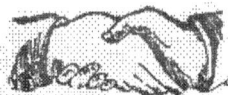

STUDENTS OF PHARMACY, we greet you. Here is our hand—SHAKE! We know your toils and pains, and would gladly aid you in your difficult vocation. Here is a little volume for you. It originated from a list of questions prepared and circulated by a class of Pharmics who were striving to hunt out the technicalities from the leading authors as a preparation for a State Examination. The questions enabled all of them to pass the State Board, and now these questions, together with many others, are tendered to you.

Our only apology for thus playing the author is that even a child may ask questions that a philosopher cannot answer. Rest assured, we shall be content to be the inquisitive child until you become the philosopher by learning to answer all of the questions we shall ask. Hoping for such splendid results, we commend this, our pride, to our Pharmic friends and trust them for the rest.

THE AUTHORS.

Ada, Ohio, June 1, 1896.

Introduction.

No subject is more intricate than Pharmacy and its attendant branches. No profession crowds the memory with a greater array of technicalities, not grouped together by logical relations so as to aid the memory, but disconnected so as the rather to confuse it. Many of these technicalities are required to be fresh in the mind for examination alone, then to be forgotten till called for by another. Even the pharmacist of long experience, if required to pass a State Board, will find it necessary to recall these forgotten subtleties, as well as to review the more important principles.

To search out these intricacies again from large volumes, perhaps, too, to overlook many, is a painful task from which the sanction of his better judgment will turn away in distaste to embrace this Quizzer with joy. Besides, a complete list of questions will afford the student a thorough review, will suggest general principles connected with each topic, will call out the technical points which the closest reader is likely to overlook on a first reading, and will serve, by well-directed questions, to focalize all these upon his memory.

The Quiz Method is the only way to get the principles of Pharmacy. You may read volume after volume and hear lecture after lecture, but if you don't get down to the technicalities by means of a quiz, you will find yourself poorly prepared for examination or practice. The Socratic Method of teaching is old, but venerable for its age, for all the so-called *new* methods of teaching that have been successful are so mainly because of the retention of the Socratic Method.

Reverencing this fact, the authors have ably applied this time-honored method to the subject of Pharmacy. This Quizzer supplements without supplanting the text-book, and thus fills a long felt want.

J. GAI SMITH.

Pharmacy.

For a Hasty Review take the * Questions.

1. *Define Pharmacy.
   Pharmacy is the science which treats of medicinal substances.

2. *Into what two chief classes may Pharmacy be divided?
   Theoretical Pharmacy and Practical Pharmacy.

3. *What is Materia Medica?
   That branch of medical science which treats of the substances used in the cure of disease.

4. *Define Magistral Pharmacy.
   Magistral, or Extemporaneous, Pharmacy treats of the preparation and dispensing of medicines intended to meet the occasion.

5. *Define Galenical Pharmacy.
   Galenical Pharmacy treats of the preparations which are made in advance and kept on hand ready for use.

6. *What is a Pharmacopœia?
   A book containing a list of medicinal substances, with descriptions, tests and formulas, selected by some recognized authority.

7. How many titles in the U. S. P.?
   989.

8. What is Metrology?
   The science which treats of weights and measures.

9. What is Weight?

The measure of the gravitating force of a body.

10. What is Volume?

Volume is the space occupied by a certain amount of matter.

11. *What weights and measures are of especial interest to the Pharmacist?

Apothecary's weight, Avoirdupois weight, Apothecary's or wine measure, and the Metric weights and measures.

12. *What is the unit of weight of the Troy and Avoirdupois weights?

The grain.

13. *How many grains in the Avoirdupois pound?

7,000.

14. *How many grains in the Avoirdupois ounce?

437.5.

15. *How many grains in the Troy pound?

5,760.

16. *How many grains in the Troy ounce?

480.

17. How many grains in a fluid ounce of water?

455.7.

18. *What system of weights and measures has been adopted by the U. S. P.?

The Metric System.

19. *What is the unit of length of the Metric System?

The meter.

20. *What is the unit of capacity?

The liter.

21. *What is the unit of weight?

The gram.

22. *What is the rule for converting the weights and measures in ordinary use into Metric weights and measures?

Multiply the quantities by the corresponding metric equivalent.

23. *How many inches in one meter?

39.37.

24. *How many cubic centimeters in one liter?

1,000.

25. *How many grains in one gram?

15.432.

26. *What is the rule for converting grams to grains?

Multiply the number of grams by 15.43.

27. *What is the rule for converting drachms to cubic centimeters?

Multiply the number of drachms by 3.75.

28. *What is the equivalent of one grain in the Metric System?

.064 m. g.

29. *What is Specific Gravity?

Specific Gravity is the weight of one body compared with the weight of an equal bulk of another body selected as the standard, both bodies having the same temperature.

30. *What is the rule for taking the specific gravity of a body heavier than water and insoluble in it?

Weigh the body in air, then weigh it in water. Divide the weight in air by the weight of water displaced. The quotient will be the specific gravity

31. *How would you take the specific gravity of a liquid?

By the specific gravity bottle, or the hydrometer.

32. What is Heat?

Heat is molecular motion.

33. Why is illuminating gas best for generating heat for pharmaceutical operations?

It is cheap, furnishes a clean, smokeless flame. The supply is constant and under perfect control.

34. *How is heat measured?

By the thermometer.

35. *What is the official thermometer?

The Centigrade.

36. Give freezing and boiling points of water on the Centigrade thermometer.

Freezing, 0°. Boiling, 100°.

37. What is the freezing point of water on the Fahrenheit thermometer?

32°.

38. What is the boiling point?

212°.

39. What is the freezing point of mercury?

40°F.

40. *How would you measure temperature below that point?

By the alcohol thermometer.

41. *What is the rule for converting Fahrenheit degrees into those of Centigrade?

Subtract 32 and divide by 1.8.

42. *What is the rule for converting Centigrade degrees into those of Fahrenheit?

Multiply by 1.8 and add 32.

43. *How many processes in Pharmacy require the use of a high heat?

Eight.

44. *Define Ignition.

Ignition is the process of strongly heating solids or semi-solids, the residue left being the object sought.

45. *What is Carbonization?

It is the process of heating organic substances without exposure to air until the volatile products are driven off and the residue has the appearance of charcoal.

46. *What is Incineration?

The process of heating organic substances with access of air until the carbon is consumed, the ashes being the object sought.

47. *What is Calcination?

It is the process of separating volatile substances from fixed inorganic matter by the application of heat without fusion.

48. *What is Fusion?

The process of liquifying solid bodies by the application of heat without the use of a solvent.

49. *What is Deflagration?

The process of heating one inorganic substance with another capable of yielding oxygen; decomposition ensues accompanied by a sudden combustion.

50. *What is Sublimation?

It is the process of separating a volatile solid from one which is not volatile by the application of heat.

51. *What is Torrefaction?

It is the process whereby organic substances have some of their constituents modified by the application of a degree of heat somewhat less than would be necessary to carbonize them.

52. *What is Vaporization?

It is the process of separating a volatile substance from a fixed or less volatile substance by the action of heat at varying temperatures.

53. What is vaporization called when used to separate volatile liquids from less volatile?

Evaporation.

54. *What name is applied to it when the volatile liquid is the object sought?

Distillation.

55. *When it is used to separate a volatile solid from another body, what is it called?

Sublimation.

56, Name two methods of increasing the rapidity of evaporation.

By increasing the temperature. By increasing the extent of surface exposed to the air.

57. What is the boiling point of a liquid?

The temperature at which it boils.

58. *Define Distillation.

Distillation is the process of vaporizing a liquid by the application of heat and recondensing the vapor.

59. *What are the objects of sublimation?

To purify volatile solids. To collect volatile solids resulting from chemical reaction at high temperatures.

60. *How would you form Cake Sublimates?

By conveying the vapors into a chamber, the temperature of which is but little below the condensing point of the substance.

61. *How are Powder Sublimates made?

By conveying the vapors into a chamber where there is a marked difference between the temperature of the air and the condensing point of the substance.

62. What is Comminution?

The process of reducing drugs to fine particles.

63. *What is Desiccation?

The process of depriving solid substances of moisture at a low temperature.

64. What are the objects of desiccation?

To facilitate comminution.
To reduce the bulk.
To aid in preservation.

65. What is Levigation?

The process of reducing substances to a state of minute division by triturating them after they have been made into paste with water or other liquid.

66. *What is Elutriation?

It is the process of obtaining a substance in fine powder by suspending an insoluble powder in water, allowing the heavier particles to fall to the bottom and decanting off the liquid containing the light particles.

67. *What is Solution?

Solution is the process whereby any substance is made to liquify or disappear when brought in contact with a solvent.

68. What effect has simple solution on temperature?

It lowers it.

69. What kind of solution would have the opposite effect?

Chemical.

70. *What is Filtration?

Filtration is the process of separating liquids from solids with the object of obtaining the liquid in a transparent condition.

71. *Distinguish between Clarification and Decoloration.

Clarification is the process of separating from liquids, without the use of filters, solid substances which interfere with their transparency.

Decoloration is the process of depriving liquids or solids in solution of color by the use of animal charcoal.

72. *Name five ways of clarifying liquids.

By the application of heat.
By increasing the fluidity of the liquid.
By the use of albumen.
By the use of milk.
By fermentation.

73. Name two good methods of separating immiscrible liquids.

By the use of the separating funnel.
By the use of the pipette.

74. *Define Precipitation.

Precipitation is the process of separating solid particles from a solution by heat, light or chemical reaction.

75. *What are the objects of precipitation?

To obtain solid substances in the form of fine powder. To effect the purification of solids. Used largely in chemical testing.

76. What is a Magma?

A thick precipitate left after the liquid is decanted.

77. How would you obtain a light precipitate?

Use cold, dilute solutions.

78. How would you obtain a heavy precipitate?

Use hot, dense solutions.

79. *How would you cause a precipitate to form in a liquid that contained albumen?

Heat it.

80. *State how you would detannate a solution by precipitation.

By the use of gelatine or ferric hydrate.

81. *What is Crystallization?

It is the process whereby substances are caused to assume certain determinate forms called crystals.

82. How would you proceed to procure crystals from a dilute solution of a crystallizable substance?

Evaporate until a pelicle forms on the surface. The substance will then crystallize.

83. What name has been given to the water that combines with a crystal?

Water of crystallization.

84. *How is water of crystallization defined?

As solid water in a combined form.

85. *What is Efflorescence?

A salt is said to effloresce when it looses its water of crystallization and turns white when brought in contact with the air.

86. *What is a Deliquescent substance?

A substance that absorbs moisture from the air and liquifies.

87. By what process are crystals deprived of their

water of crystallization?

By exsiccation.

88. *What is Dialysis?

The process of separating crystallizable from non-crystallizable substances by placing a solution containing both on a porous diaphragm
the under side of which is in contact with water.

89. Define Crystalloids.

Crystalloids are substances which always have the crystalline form.

90. Define Colloids.

Colloids are substances which never crystallize.

91. *How does Extraction differ from Solution?

Extraction differs from solution in the fact that the presence of insoluble matter is implied in the former, and the soluble constituents
must be extracted by appropriate methods.

92. *Name five methods of extraction.

1. Maceration and expression. 2. Percolation. 3. Digestion. 4. Infusion. 5. Decoction.

93. *How does Digestion differ from Maceration?

Digestion requires the use of heat. Maceration does not require the
use of heat.

94. How does Expression differ from Extraction?

Expression is the forcible extraction of liquids from solids.

95. *What is Percolation?

Percolation is the process of depriving a powder, contained in a per-
colator, of its soluble constituents by the descent of a solvent
through it.

96. In the process of percolation how can we tell when
the drug is exhausted?

Absence of color or taste is evidence of exhaustion.

97. *What two important classes of preparations are made largely by percolation?

    1. Tinctures. 2. Fluid extracts.

AQUÆ—Waters.

98. *What are official waters?

    They are aqueous solutions of volatile substances.

99. How many forms of matter are used in the preparation of waters?

    Three: solid, liquid and gaseous.

100. By how many methods are they prepared?

    Five.

101. *Name three methods.

    1. Simple solution in cold water. 2. Gaseous solution. 3. Distillation.

102. Name two made by distillation.

    1. Aqua Destillata. 2. Aqua Rosae Fortior.

103. *Name two that are made by gaseous solution, with strength.

    1. Aqua Ammonia, 10 per cent. 2. Aqua Chlori, .4 per cent.

104. What water is made by the solution of a volatile solid?

    Aqua Camphorae.

105. *Give the U. S. P. definition of Aqua Hydrogenii Dioxidi.

    A slightly acid aqueous solution of Hydrogen Dioxide, containing, when freshly prepared, about 3 per cent of the pure dioxide, corresponding to about ten volumes of available oxygen.

106. *How is Aqua Chlori prepared?
By dissolving chlorine gas in water.

SYRUPI—Syrups.

107. What are Syrups?
Syrups are concentrated solutions of sugar in aqueous liquids.

108. By how many methods are they prepared?
Five.

109. *Name three methods.
1. By agitation without heat. 2. By the addition of the medicating substance to syrup. 3. By digestion.

110. What syrup is made from an aromatic tincture?
Aromatic Syrup of Rhubarb.

111. *What syrup contains ammonia water? Why?
Syrup of Senega.
To dissolve the pectin.

112. Name a syrup that contains three fluid extracts.
Compound Syrup Sarsaparilla.

113. *How is Syrup of Ferrous Iodide made? How should it be kept? Why?
Made by acting on iron wire with iodine and water. When the solution becomes green it is filtered into syrup.
Should be kept in small well-stoppered and completely filled bottles exposed to the light. (*Remington.*)
To prevent the liberation of free iodine. Strength, 10 per cent.

114. *Why is Syrup of Wild Cherry made by the cold process?
To prevent the loss of Hydrocyanic Acid.

115. What are the ingredients in Syrup of Hydriodic Acid, and strength?

Potassium Iodide.
Potassium Hypophosphite.
Tartaric Acid.
Water.
Diluted Alcohol.
Contains one per cent, by weight, of absolute hydriodic acid.

116. What syrup is made by maceration?

Syrup of Tar.

117. Name a syrup made by digestion.

Syrup of Tolu.

118. *Name four syrups that contain acid.

1. Syrup of Citric Acid. 2. Syrup of Ipecac. 3. Syrup of Garlic. 4. Syrup of Squill.

119. *What syrup contains Potassium Carbonate?

Syrup of Rhubarb.

120. *What is the official name for Easton's Syrup?

Syrupus Ferri, Quininae et Strychninae Phosphatum.

121. *Would you use fresh or dried peel in the preparation of Syrup of Orange?

Fresh.

___

MELLITA—Honeys.

122. *What is the official name for Honeys?

Mellita.

123. How many are official?

Three.

124. *How do they differ from syrups?

2 b

They differ merely in the use of honey as a base instead of syrup.

125. *What is the official name for Clarified Honey? How is it prepared?

Mel Despumatum.
Heat the honey mixed with paper pulp. Strain and add five per cent of glycerin.

126. What are the ingredients in Mel Rosæ?

Clarified honey, fluid extract of rose.

MUCILAGINES—Mucilages.

127. *What are Mucilages?

They are thick, adhesive liquids made by dissolving gum in water.

128. How many are official?

Four.

129. What two are made by the cold process?

Mucilage of acacia, mucilage of sassafras pith.

130. *What mucilages must be freshly prepared when wanted?

Mucilage of sassafras pith and mucilage of elm.

131. How is Mucilage of Acacia directed to be kept?

In well-stoppered and completely filled bottles in a cool place

132. Why is Mucilage of Tragacanth directed to be strained forcibly through muslin?

Only a part of the tragacanth dissolves, the remainder only swells up and it must be forced through the strainer.
Note.—Mucilages can be used as an antidote for all corrosive poisons.

EMULSA—Emulsions.

133. *Define Emulsions.

They are aqueous liquids in which oleaginous substances are suspended by the use of gum or other viscid matter.

134. How many are official?

Four.

135. *Into how many classes are emulsions divided? Name them.

Two.
Natural emulsions and prepared emulsions.

136. What are Natural Emulsions?

Emulsions that exist naturally, as milk, yolk of egg.

137. What are Manufactured Emulsions?

Those which are made artificially.

138. *How are Gum Resin emulsions made?

By triturating the gum resin with water.

139. *How are Seed Emulsions made?

By triturating the seeds with water.

140. *What seed emulsion is official?

Emulsion of Almond.

141. What is Emulsion of Chloroform?

A tragacanth emulsion.

142. How would you prepare an Emulsion of Pepo?

Triturate the seeds with water.

143. How would you make an emulsion of a volatile oil?

Mix the volatile oil with a fixed oil and proceed in the usual way.

144. *Give general formula for emulsions.

Oil four parts, water two parts, gum one part. Form the nucleus and dilute to the required amount.

MISTURÆ—Mixtures.

145. *What are Mixtures?

They are simply mechanical mixtures of insoluble medicinal substances in aqueous liquids.

146. How many are official?

Four.

147. How many contain an insoluble powder?

Three.

148. What are the ingredients in Mistura Rhei et Sodae?

Sodium Bicarbonate.
Fluid Extract of Rhubarb.
Fluid Extract of Ipecac.
Glycerin.
Spirit of Peppermint.
Water.

149. *What is the official name for Brown Mixture?

Mistura Glycyrrhizae Composita.

150. What form of Glycyrrhiza does it contain?

The pure Extract of Glycyrrhiza.

151. What salt of iron does Griffith's Mixture contain?

Ferrous Carbonate.

152. What mixture contains a Wine, a Tincture, a Spirit and an Extract?

Mistura Glycyrrhizae Composita.

GLYCERITA—Glycerites.

153. Define Glycerites.

Glycerites are mixtures of medicinal substances with glycerin.

154. What is their chief advantage?

The ease with which they can be diluted with water or alcohol without precipitation is their chief advantage.

155. How many are official?

Six.

156. *How many old ones and how many new ones were added to the U. S. P. of 1890?

Two old ones and two new ones.

157. *Name one that is used internally, with the dose.

Glycerite of Carbolic Acid. Dose, 5 m.

158. What alkaloid is precipitated by Glycerite of Hydrastis?

Berberine.

_____

SPIRITUS—Spirits.

159. *What are Spirits?

Alcoholic solutions of volatile substances.

160. How many are official, and by how many methods are they prepared?

Twenty-five. Five.

161. Name three ways of making Spirits.

Maceration. Distillation. Chemical reaction.

162. Name a spirit made by the solution of a volatile solid.

Spirit of Camphor.

163. *What change was made in the formula of Spirits of Camphor in the U. S. P. 1890?

The water was omitted.

164. *What three spirits are made by solution with

maceration?

Spirit of Lemon. Spirit of Peppermint. Spirit of Spearmint.

165. *What general synonym has been given to the spirits made by maceration?

Essences.

166. What is Spiritus Glonoini?

An alcoholic solution of Nitroglycerin containing 1 per cent. by weight, of the active ingredient.

167. *What spirit is made by chemical reaction?

Spirit of Nitrous Ether.

168. What two spirits are made by distillation?

Spiritus Frumenti. Spiritus vini Gallici.

169. *How old must the spirits made by distillation be before being used?   .

Whiskey, two years. Brandy, four years.

170. *How is Spiritus Ammoniae made?

By heating stronger water of ammonia to drive off the gas, and re-dissolving the gas in alcohol.

171. *What spirit was made official to make an elixir, and what kind of alcohol does it contain?

Spirit of Phosphorus. Absolute Alcohol.

172. *Why do you use ammonia water in Aromatic Spirits of Ammonia.

To neutralize the Ammonium Bicarbonate.

COLLODIA—Collodions.

173. *What are Collodions?

Liquid preparations having for their base a solution of pyroxylin in a mixture of alcohol and ether.

174. How are they applied? For what purpose?

They are applied with a brush. For the purpose of acting as a protective or to bring a medicating substance in contact with the skin.

175. *What are the ingredients in Collodium Stypticum?

Tannic Acid.
Alcohol.
Ether.
Collodion.

176. *What are the ingredients in Collodium Fexile?

Collodion.
Canada Turpentine.
Castor Oil.

LINIMENTA—Liniments.

177. *What are Liniments?

They are solutions or mixtures of various substances in oily or alcoholic liquids.

178. How are liniments intended to be applied?

They are to be applied externally by friction and rubbing of the skin.

179. How many are official?

Nine.

180. *What one is a soluble soap?

Liniment of Ammonia.

181. *What one is an insoluble soap?

Lime Liniment.

182. What are the ingredients in Linimentum Bella-

donnae?

Fluid Extract of Belladonna.　Camphor.

183. What two contain a form of soap?

Linimentum Saponis, Linimentum Saponis Mollis.

184. What are the ingredients in Compound Liniment
of Mustard?

Volatile Oil of Mustard.
Fluid Extract of Mezereum.
Castor Oil.
Camphor.
Alcohol.

185. What are the ingredients in Chloroform Liniment?

Soap Liniment.
Chloroform.

INFUSA—Infusions.

186. *What are Infusions?

Liquid preparations made by treating vegetable substances with hot
or cold water.

187. *By how many methods are they prepared?
Name them.

Four.　By maceration, by digestion, by percolation, by diluting
fluid extracts.

188. Which process is most frequently used?

Maceration.

189. *What is the chief objection to making infusions
by diluting fluid extracts?

When an alcoholic fluid extract is diluted to the extent necessary to
make an infusion it causes serious precipitation.

190. *In making infusions which would you use and

why, a coarse or fine powder?

Coarse powder; a fine powder would be hard to separate from the liquid.

191. What infusions are made by Maceration?

Infusion of Digitalis, Compound Infusion of Senna.

192. *What are the ingredients in Compound Infusion of Senna?

Senna.
Manna.
Magnesium Sulphate.
Fennel, bruised.
Boiling water.
Cold water.

193. *In the preparation of Infusion of Digitalis, why not add the cinnamon water and the alcohol while the solution is hot?

The heat would cause them to volatilize and escape.

194. *For what purpose is Aromatic Sulphuric Acid used in Infusion of Cinchona?

To dissolve the alkaloids.

195. Why not make Infusion of Wild Cherry by digestion?

The heat would cause the hydrocyanic acid to escape.

196. *How do Decoctions differ from Infusions?

Decoctions are made by boiling, Infusions are made with either hot or cold water.

197. How do the two official Decoctions differ in the method of preparation?

Decoction of Cetraria is made by boiling for a short time, then throwing the water away and using fresh water; this is done to remove

the bitter principle. In the preparation of Compound Decoction
of Sarsaparilla, the drug is exhausted with the first water used.

TINCTURÆ—Tinctures.

198. *What are Tinctures?

Alcoholic solutions of non-volatile substances.

199. What exception to the rule?

Tincture of Iodine.

200. *How many tinctures are official?

Seventy-two.

201. *In what different ways are they prepared?

By maceration, by percolation, by solution or dilution.

202. *What is used as a menstruum?

Alcohol, Diluted Alcohol of various strengths, Aromatic Spirits of
Ammonia, mixtures of Alcohol, Water and Glycerin.

203. *What advantage have they over Infusions and
Decoctions?

They are permanent preparations and can be kept on hand ready
for use.

204. *What is their chief advantage over fluid extracts?

They can be added to aqueous liquids without serious precipitation.

205. Why is glycerin used in some tinctures?

To hold the tannin in solution.

206. Are tinctures of uniform strength?

No.

207. *What substances are directed to be macerated
when used in making tinctures?

Resins, balsams, gums, etc.

208. *Name a tincture made by simple solution and one made by dilution.

Tincture of Iodine, by solution.
Tincture of Ferric Chloride, by dilution.

209. What is the strength of the following tinctures?

Tr. Aconite, 35 per cent. Tr. Cinchona, 20 per cent. Tr. Veratrum Virides, 40 per cent. Tr. Aloes, 30 per cent. Tr. Hyoscyamus, 15 per cent. Tr. Rhubarb, 12 per cent. Tr. Opium, 10 per cent. Tr. Iodine, 7 per cent. Tr. Cantharides, 5 per cent. Tr. Opium Camphorated, 1.6 per cent.

210. *What tincture is made from an extract?

Tincture of Nux Vomica.

211. Name three tinctures that contain purified Aloes.

Tincture of Aloes. Tincture of Aloes and Myrrh. Compound Tincture of Benzoin.

212. Name two tinctures that contain Licorice root.

Tincture of Aloes. Tincture of Aloes and Myrrh.

213. *What tinctures are made with Aromatic Spirits of Ammonia?

Ammoniated Tincture of Guaiac. Ammoniated Tincture of Valerian.

214. *In the preparation of what tincture is Benzin used?

Tincture of Lactucarium.

VINA MEDICATA—Medicated Wines.

215. *What are Medicated Wines?

Liquid preparations containing the soluble principles of medicinal substances dissolved in wine.

216. What class of preparations do they resemble, and

what is the chief difference?

They resemble tinctures, differing merely in the character of the menstruum.

217. *What does the U. S. P. direct to be added to white wine when used as a menstruum?

Alcohol or an alcoholic tincture.

218. *How many of the official wines are medicated?

Eight.

219. *What should be the alcoholic strength of the non-medicated wines?

10 to 14 per cent.

220. Name two wines made by maceration.

Wine of Colchicum Seed. Wine of Opium.

221. Name two wines made by percolation.

Wine of Colchicum Root. Wine of Ergot.

222. What are the ingredients in Wine of Opium?

Powdered Opium.
Cassia Cinnamon.
Cloves.
Alcohol.
White Wine.

223. *Why is boiling water directed to be used in Wine of Antimony?

To dissolve the Tartar Emetic.

EXTRACTA FLUIDA—Fluid Extracts.

224. *What are Fluid Extracts?

Fluid Extracts are alcoholic liquid preparations, one cubic centimeter of which represents the medicinal virtues of one gram of the drug.

225. In what other way could they be defined?

As concentrated tinctures.

226. *How many are official?

Eighty-eight.

227. *What are their chief advantages?

Permanency, Concentration. The relation of gram to cubic centimeter.

228. *How are they prepared?

By percolation with partial evaporation. (Official.)
By percolation with incomplete exhaustion.
By repercolation.
By vacuum maceration with percolation.

229. *How is permanence secured?

By the use of alcoholic menstrua.

230. How many Fluid Extracts contain glycerin, and what is it used for?

Sixteen contain glycerin. Used to prevent precipitation.

231. *For what purpose is Acetic Acid used in Fluid Extract of Conium?

Used to fix the alkaloid "Conine".

232. Of what use is the acid in Fluid Extract of Ergot?

Used to fix the alkaloids.

233. *Why is Acetic Acid used in Fluid Extract of Sanguinaria?

Used to prevent precipitation.

234. *What alkaloids are dissolved by the Acetic Acid

in Fluid Extract of Nux Vomica?

Strychnine and brucine.

235. Why is Ammonia water used in Fluid Extract of Senega?

Used to dissolve the Pectin.

236. *Why is Ammonia Water used in Fluid Extract of Glycyrrhiza?

To dissolve the glycyrrhizin.

237. What compound Fluid Extract is official?

Compound Fluid Extract of Sarsaparilla.

238. What Fluid Extract is made from Aromatic Powder?

Aromatic Fluid Extract.

239. *What Fluid Extract is made with boiling water and Alcohol added to preserve?

Fluid Extract of Triticum.

240. *What Fluid Extract is made with boiling water and Alcohol and Glycerin added to preserve?

Fluid Extract of Castanea.

241. *What Fluid Extract is standardized, and what per cent. of alkaloids must it contain?

Fluid Extract of Nux Vomica. Must contain 1.5 per cent. of alkaloids.

EXTRACTA—Extracts.

242. *What are Extracts?

Extracts are solid or semi-solid preparations made by evaporating solutions of vegetable substances.

243. How many are official?

Thirty-three.

244. *How are they prepared?

By maceration with percolation and evaporation. By expression with evaporation.

245. *What menstrua are used?

Water, alcohol, diluted alcohol of various strengths, acetic acid, ether, and diluted solutions of ammonia.

246. *What two Extracts contain Acetic Acid? Why is the acid used?

Extract of Nux Vomica. Extract of Colchicum Root.
Used to dissolve the alkaloids.

247. *What per cent of alkaloids must Extract of Nux Vomica contain?

15 per cent.

248. *How much Morphine must Extract of Opium contain?

18 per cent.

249. *What are the U. S. P. requirements of Extract of Glycyrrhiza.

It must contain 60 per cent of soluble matter.

250. What two Extracts contain Sugar of Milk? For what purpose?

Extract of Nux Vomica. Extract of Opium.
Used as a diluent so that the finished extracts shall contain the proper percentage of alkaloids.

251. *In the preparation of what Extract is Ammonia Water used, and why?

Pure Extract of Glycyrrhiza.

To dissolve the glycyrrhizin.

252. What Extract is made from a fluid extract?

Extract of Ergot.

253. What Extract is largely used as a pill excipient?

Extract of Gentian.

254. What is the official name and the ingredients in the only compound extract?

Extractum Colocynthidis Compositum.
Extract of Colocynth.
Purified Aloes.
Cardamom.
Resin of Scammony.
Soap.
Alcohol.

255. *What may be added to extracts to prevent them from becoming hard?

Glycerin.

256. *What Extract is made from an inspissated juice?

Extract of Taraxacum.

257. How may Extracts be made without the use of heat?

By freezing the juices, then expressing them, and drying the concentrated juice in the sun.

258. *What is the chief objection to extracts?

Their variable strength.

OLEORESINÆ—Oleoresins.

259. *What are Oleoresins?

They are liquid preparations consisting principally of natural oils and resins extracted from vegetable substances by percolation with ether.

260. *Are they identical with fluid extracts? If not, why?

They are not; They bear no uniform relation to the drug. The menstruum used extracts principles which are often insoluble in alcohol.

261. How do they differ from all other liquid prepara-rations?

They are without exception the most concentrated liquid prepara-tions that are produced.

262. *How do Oleoresin of Aspedium and Oleoresin of Cubeb differ when kept on hand?

A precipitate forms in Oleoresin of Aspedium which must be shaken up and dispensed with the liquid part. The precipitate in Oleore-sin of Cubeb is inert and should be filtered out.

ACETA—Vinegars.

263. *What are Vinegars.

Vinegars are solutions of the active principles of drugs in diluted acetic acid.

264. *How many are official, and what is the strength of each?

Two. Each represents the strength of 10 per cent. of the drug.

265. What are the ingredients in Acetum Opii?

Powdered Opium.
Nutmeg.
Sugar.
Diluted Acetic Acid.

266. *What is their chief advantages over tinctures?

They can be added to aqueous liquids without serious precipitation,

3 C

RESINA—Resins.

267. What are Resins?   How many official?

Resins are solid preparations consisting principally of the resinous principles from vegetable bodies. Five are official.

268. *How do they differ from extracts?

They contain only those principles which are soluble in alcohol and insoluble in water. Extracts contain the principles that are soluble in both alcohol and water.

269. How are they prepared?

Two are obtained as a by-product from the distillation of volatile oils. Three are made by adding an alcoholic solution of a resinous drug to water, and collecting and drying the precipitate.

270. *Why is Hydrochloric Acid used in Resin of Podophyllin?

Used to facilitate precipitation.

GUMS.

271. *What are Gums?

Gums are vegetable substances insoluble in alcohol, but with water they form a thick glutinous liquid, mucilage.

272. *What three proximate principles are found in gums?

(a) Arabin, a soluble gum found in tragacanth.
(b) Bassorin, an insoluble gum found in tragacanth.
(c) Cerasin, an insoluble gum found in cherry gum.

273. How do gums differ from starch or cellulin?

They differ from starch or cellulin by being soluble in water or swelling up when in contact with it.

274. How do gums differ from sugars?

Gums differ from sugars by being incapable of vinous fermentation with yeast.

SUGARS.

275. *What are Sugars?

Sugars are organic bodies having a sweet taste, generally of vegetable origin, crystallizable, soluble in water and only slightly soluble in alcohol.

276. *Into what two classes are sugars divided?

Fermentable and non-fermentable.

277. Which is the more important class?

The fermentable sugars are the more important.

278. *Into what two sub-classes are the fermentable sugars divided?

(a) Glucoses, or sugars directly subject to vinous fermentation.
(b) Saccharoses, or sugars indirectly subject to vinous fermentation.

SOAPS.

279. *What are Soaps chemically?

Chemically, soaps are oleates.

280. *Into how many classes are soaps divided? Name them.

Two. Soluble and insoluble.

281. Name two insoluble soaps used in Pharmacy.

Lead Plaster and Lime Liniment.

282. What are the official preparations of soap?

Soap Plaster and Soap Liniment.

283. What official preparation made from Soft Soap?

Liniment of Soft Soap.

284. *How are Hard Soaps made?

Soaps are made hard by using a fat that contains much stearin and soda for the alkali.

285. *How are Soft Soaps made?

Soft soaps are made by using a fat that contains a large proportion of olein and potassa for the alkali.

VOLATILE OILS.

286. *What are Volatile Oils?

Volatile oils are volatile odorous principles which produce a greasy stain that disappears on the application of heat.

287. *Into what classes are they divided?

(a) Terpenes.
(b) Oxygenated Oils.
(c) Sulphurated Oils.
(d) Nitrogenated Oils.

288. *What are the proximate constituents of Volatile Oils?

Volatile oils consist of two principles, Stearopten the solid portion, and Eleopten the liquid portion.

289. *How can the stearoptens be separated from the liquid portion?

When stearopten and eleopten congeal at different temperatures they may be separated by compressing the frozen oil between folds of bibulous paper; the liquid portion is absorbed by the paper while the solid part remains between the folds.

290. What are the best solvents for volatile oils, and to what extent are they soluble in water?

Alcohol, Ether and Chloroform are the best solvents. They are only soluble in water to the extent of one or two parts to a thousand.

291. *What effect has exposure to light and air upon volatile oils?

It injures the quality and destroys the fragrance of volatile oils. Ozone is developed, and they thicken and become resinified.

292. *What are the chief adulterants of volatile oils and the test for each?

(a) Fixed Oils. Detected by adding the oil to the filter paper and applying heat; if the oil is pure the stain will disappear, but if it contains a fixed oil the stain will be permanent.

(b) Alcohol. Detected by adding iodine and potassium bicarbonate to the oil; if alcohol is present iodoform will be formed.

(c) Chloroform. When distilled at 60°C. the distillate should not have any of the properties of chloroform.

(d) Synthetic Oils. Detected by the odor.

293. What is the chief method of obtaining volatile oils?

By distillation with water.

294. What is Eufleurage?

Eufleurage is a process used for extracting the odors of very delicate flowers, by sprinkling the flowers on a thin layer of fat, allowing them to stand until the fat has absorbed the odor. The volatile products may then be obtained by macerating the fat in alcohol.

295. *Name the official Stearoptens.

Menthol, Thymol and Camphor.

FIXED OILS AND FATS.

296. *What are Fixed Oils and Fats?

Fixed oils and fats are oily substances obtained from both the animal and vegetable kingdom. They are greasy to the touch, produce a greasy stain on paper which does not disappear on the application of heat.

297. *What are Fixed Oils and Fats chemically?

Chemically, they are compound ethers of higher members of the fatty acids.

298. How may rancid oils be purified?

They can, usually, be purified by shaking them with hot water, then with a cold solution of sodium carbonate, then washing them with cold water.

299. *What are the proximate principles of Fixed Oils?

Olein, the liquid portion.
Palmitin and Stearin are both solid.

300. How is the Olein separated from the solid parts?

By freezing the oil and then subjecting it to hydraulic pressure; the liquid part is forced out while the solid portions remain in the press.

301. What is their chief use in Pharmacy?

To form soaps and as a base for ointments.

EMPLASTRA—Plasters.

302. *What are Plasters?

Plasters are substances intended for external application, of such a consistence that they adhere to the skin and require the aid of heat in spreading them.

303. What is the basis of most plasters?

Either Lead Plaster, a gum-resin or Burgundy pitch.

304. *When spread plasters become hard on the surface, how may they be made to adhere to the skin?

By brushing the surface with tincture of camphor.

305. Would you use a high heat in the preparation of plasters, and why?

No. A high heat may cause decomposition and the loss of any volatile constituents that the substance may contain.

306. *Give full Latin title for Warming Plaster.

Emplastrum Picis Cantharidatum.

307. Give full Latin title for Diachylon Plaster.

Emplastrum Plumbi.

308. Give the Latin title and ingredients in Adhesive Plaster.

Emplastrum Resinæ.
    Resin.
    Yellow Wax.
    Lead Plaster.

309. *What useful by-product is produced in the manufacture of Lead Plaster?

Glycerin.

310. *What are the ingredients in Emplastrum Ammoniaci Cum Hydrargyro? What per cent. of mercury? •

Ammoniac.
Mercury.
Oleate of Mercury.
Diluted Acetic Acid.
Lead Plaster.
Contains 18 per cent of mercury.

UNGUENTA—Ointments.

311. *What are Ointments?

Ointments are fatty preparations of a softer consistence than cerates, intended to be used externally.

312. *By how many methods are Ointments prepared?
How many are official?

Three—by fusion; by incorporation; by chemical reaction. There are twenty-three official.

313. What are the ingredients in Basilicon Ointment?

Resin.
Yellow Wax.
Lard.

314. Name two ointments made by fusion.

Unguentum Aquæ Rosæ.
Unguentum Diachylon.

315. *What three maxims should be observed in dispensing ointments?

Never dispense ointments that are rancid. They should always be smooth and free from irritating particles. Ointments containing free acid or iodine should not be rubbed with an iron or steel spatula.

316. *Name two ointments that should not be made with an iron or steel spatula.

Unguentum Hydrargyri Nitratis.
Unguentum Iodi.

317. Why is Potassium Iodide used in Unguentum Iodi?

To dissolve the iodine.

318. *Why is Sodium Hyposulphite used in Unguentum Potassii Iodidi?

To decolorize any iodine that may be liberated from the potassium iodide.

319. What Ointment contains Castor Oil?

Unguentum Hydrargyri Oxidi Rubri.

320. *What chemical change takes place in the preparation of Citrine Ointment?

The olein of the oil is converted into elaidin.

321. What per cent. of mercury in Blue Ointment?

50 per cent.

_____

CERATA—Cerates.

322. *What are Cerates?

Cerates are unctious substances of such a consistence that they may
be easily spread with a spatula without the aid of heat.

323. *By how many methods are they prepared? How
many are official?

Two—fusion; incorporation. Six cerates are official.

324. *How do they differ from ointments?

They are of a harder consistence than ointments. They all contain
wax to raise the melting point.

325. What is the official name for Goulard's Cerate?
By what process is it made?

Ceratum Plumbi Subacetatis.
It is the only official cerate made by incorporation.

326. What are the ingredients in Ceratum Cantharidis?

Cantharides.
Yellow Wax.
Resin.
Lard.
Oil of Turpentine.

_____

CHARTÆ—Papers.

327. *Name the official Chartæ.

Charta Potassi Nitratis.
Charta Sinapis.

328. *Give the ingredients of Charta Sinapis.

Black Mustard.
India Rubber.
Benzin.
Carbon Disulphide.

———

PILULÆ—Pills.

329. *What are pills?

Pills are small solid bodies, generally of a globular or lenticular
shape, which are intended to be swallowed to produce medication.

330. *Of what does a pill mass consist?

The active ingredients and the excipient.

331. *What are the essential requirements of a pill
mass?

It must be adhesive, firm and plastic.   •

332. When would you use Confection of Rose for an
excipient?

When the amount of the active ingredient is small and dilution is
necessary.

333. *What makes a good excipient for volatile oils?

Magnesia or Soap.

334. *What excipient would you use for oxidizable
substances, such as Potassium Permanganate
and Silver Nitrate?

Vaseline or Cacao Butter.

335. *What official pills are directed to be coated?

Pills of Phosphorus and Pills of Ferrous Iodide.

336. By what different names are pills of Ferrous Carbonate known?

Pilulæ Ferri Carbonatis.
Ferruginous Pills.
Blaud's Pills.

437. What is the official name of Plummer's Pills?

Pilulæ Antimonii Compositæ

438. *Give the ingredients of Compound Cathartic Pills.

Compound Extract of Colocynth.
Mild Mercurous Chloride.
Extract of Jalap.
Gamboge.
Water.

339. What are the ingredients in Vegetable Cathartic Pills.

Compound Extract of Colocynth.
Extract of Hyoscyamus.
Extract of Jalap.
Extract of Leptandra.
Resin of Podophyllin.
Oil of Peppermint.
Water.

340. *What general rule must be observed in the choice of pill excipients?

Never use an excipient alone which is a perfect solvent for the solid substance.

341. What is the strength of Phosphorus Pills?

Each pill contains .01 gr. of Phosphorus.

342. What is the strength of Opium Pills.

Each pill contains 1 gr. of Opium.

343. Pill masses are official in the U. S. P. under what title? Name all the official masses.

Massa. The official masses are—
Massa Copaibæ.
Massa Ferri Carbonatis.
Massa Hydrargyri.

PULVERES—Powders.

344. What are powders?

They are dry, medicinal substances reduced to fine particles to facilitate absorption.

345. How many powders are official?

Nine.

346. *Give the official name for Seidlitz Powder.

Pulvis Effervescens Compositus.

347. What are the ingredients in Aromatic Powder?

Ceylon Cinnamon.
Ginger.
Cardamom.
Nutmeg.

348. *Give the official name and ingredients of Tully's Powder.

Pulvis Morphiuae Compositus.
Morphine Sulphate.
Camphor.
Glycyrrhiza.
Precipitated Calcium Carbonate.
Alcohol.

349. Why is alcohol used in Tully's Powder?

To aid in powdering the camphor.

350. *Give the official name for Pulvis Purgans.

Pulvis Jalapae Compositus.

351. What are the ingredients in Pulvis Rhei Compositus?

Rhubarb.
Magnesia.
Ginger.

352. *What are the ingredients in Pulvis Glycyrrhizæ
Compositus?

Senna.
Glycyrrhiza.
Washed Sulphur.
Oil of Fennel.
Sugar.

INORGANIC ACIDS.

353. *What are the chief properties of the inorganic
acids?

They have a sour taste, all caustic and corrosive, combine with
metals to form salts, turn blue litmus paper red.

354. To what three classes of acids do they belong?

Hydracids, Oxyacids, Anhydrides.

355. Distinguish between an Oxyacid, a Hydracid and
an Anhydride.

An oxyacid contains oxygen; as HNO_3.
A hydracid contains no oxygen; as HCl.
An Anhydride forms a true acid when added to water.

356. What is the strength of the official acids?

They vary from 2 to 99 per cent.

357. *What is the strength of the dilute acids?

All dilute acids are 10 per cent., except HCy, 2 per cent., Dilute Acetic Acid, 6 per cent, Dilute Nitrohydrochloric Acid, 22 per cent.

358. What acid is 99 per cent. pure?

Glacial Acetic Acid.

359. How do acids compare in weight with water?

They are all heavier than water, except Aromatic Sulphuric Acid.

360. *Into what two classes are commercial acids divided?

Chemically Pure, "C. P."
Medicinally Pure, "M. P."

361. *What is their chief use in Pharmacy?

As a solvent for metals to form salts.

362. *What are their medicinal properties?

Tonic and refrigerant.

363. What is the U. S. P. definition of Acidum Nitricum?

A liquid composed of 68 per cent. by weight of absolute Nitric Acid and 32 per cent. of water.

364. How is Aqua Regia prepared?

By mixing Nitric Acid and Hydrocloric Acid.

365. *What are the ingredients in Aromatic Sulphuric Acid?

Sulphuric Acid.
Tincture of Ginger.
Oil of Cinnamon.
Alcohol.

366. *How much acid by weight and volume does Aromatic Sulphuric Acid contain?

10 per cent. by volume, 20 per cent. by weight.

367. What is the principal use of Phosphoric Acid in Pharmacy?

To make the dilute Phosphoric Acid.

THE HALOGENS.

368. *Describe Chlorine.

Chlorine is a greenish-yellow gaseous body having a suffocating odor.

369. *What is its most useful property?

Its most useful and characteristic property is that of bleaching organic coloring matter. It is also one of the most reliable disinfectants.

370. In what combination is it used as a disinfectant?

In combination with lime as bleaching powder.

371. What is the official name of Bleaching Powder?

Calx Chlorata.

372. Describe Bromine?

Bromine is a dark red, non-metallic liquid.

373. How is it prepared?

By decomposing crude magnesium bromide with chlorine.

374. *Name two sources of Iodine.

The ashes of sea-weeds and the mother-liquors obtained from the crystallization of sodium nitrate.

375. *Is Iodine an elementary substance or a compound?

It is a non-metallic element.

SULPHUR.

376. How is Sulphur found?

Uncombined, and in the form of sulphates and sulphides.

377. *In what three forms is free sulphur official?

Sulphur Sublimatum.
Sulphur Lotum.
Sulphur Praecipitatum.

378. *Why is Ammonia Water used in preparing Washed Sulphur?

To neutralize the Sulphuric Acid which is frequently found in Sublimed Sulphur.

PHOSPHORUS.

379. *What is Phosphorus?

A non-metallic element prepared by heating acid calcium phosphate with charcoal.

380. What are the Phosphorus preparations used for?

As a tonic in defective nerve nutrition.

CARBON PREPARATIONS.

381. How is Carbo Animalis Purificatus prepared?

By boiling animal charcoal with dilute hydrochloric acid, then washing it to remove all traces of the acid.

382. What is the official test for the purity of Purified Animal Charcoal?

When boiled with a :mixture of potassium hydrate and water the filtrate should be colorless.

SILICON.

383. What official preparation is made from Silicon?

Liquor Sodii Silicatus.

384. What is its principal use?

Preparing mechanical dressings.

THE ALKALI METALS.

385. *Name the Alkali Metals.

Potassium, Sodium, Lithium and Ammonium.

386. Describe them briefly.

They have strongly marked physical and chemical properties. They combine with acids to form salts, restore the color of reddened litmus paper, change vegetable blue to green and yellow to brown. They are very soft, can be easily cut with a knife. Their specific gravity is so low that they will float upon water, but when brought in contact with it they inflame spontaneously. Hence they must be kept in a liquid that is free from oxygen.

387. Are their salts soluble or insoluble?

Soluble.

388. *Give two sources of Potassium.

The ashes from beet sugar residues, from impure potassium chloride found in the mines in Germany.

389. How many official preparations of Potassium?

Twenty-four.

4 d

390. *What is the source of Potassium Bitartrate?

Argols, a substance deposited in wine casks during the fermentation of the grape juice.

391. How would you dispense powders of Potassium Acetate?

Wrap the powder in waxed paper and then in tin-foil.

392. *Why are sodium salts more frequently used than the potassium salts?

It is largely a matter of local custom, but the sodium salts are cheaper and more soluble.

393. How is Sodium Arsenate made?

By heating together arsenous acid, sodium nitrate and sodium carbonate.

394. How many official salts of Lithium?

Six.

395. *What are the salts of Lithium used for?

Used for gout and rheumatism.

AMMONIA.

396. *What is the chief source of ammonia?

The source of nearly all the Ammonia met with in commerce is the Ammonia gas obtained in distilling coal in the manufacture of illuminating gas.

397. *Why are ammonium salts classed with those of the alkali metals?

Because they resemble them so closely in their chemical and physical properties.

398. What effect has heat on salts of Ammonium?

The salts of ammonium are completely volatilized at high temperatures.

399. *What liquid preparations of Ammonia are official?

Aqua Ammoniae, Aqua Ammoniae Fortior, Spiritus Ammoniae and Aromatic Spirits of Ammonia.

400. *State the strength of three of them.

Ammonia Water, 10 per cent.; Stronger Ammonia Water, 28 per cent.; Spirit of Ammonia, 10 per cent.

MAGNESIUM.

401. In what forms is Magnesium found in nature?

As Chloride, Sulphate and Carbonate.

402. Light magnesia is made by calcining the light magnesium carbonate. How would you prepare the heavy magnesium?

By calcining the heavy magnesium carbonate.

403. How could you reduce the bulk of light magnesia?

By triturating it.

404. *What are the ingredients in Liquor Magnesia Citratis?

Magnesium Carbonate.
Citric Acid.
Syrup of Citric Acid.
Potassium Bicarbonate.
Water.

CALCIUM.

405. How is Liquor Calcis made?

By washing lime with distilled water to remove other soluble salts; then adding more water and allowing it to stand on the lime so as to insure a saturated solution.

406. *How should it be kept? Why?

Should be kept in tightly-stoppered bottles.
To prevent the absorption of carbon dioxide which would cause the dissolved lime to precipitate as insoluble calcium carbonate.

ZINC.

407. *Give the U. S. P. definition for Zinc.

Metallic zinc, in the form of thin sheets, or irregular, granulated pieces.

408. What is the color of the precipitate when a solution of a zinc salt is treated with ammonium sulphide?

White. Zinc Sulphide.

409. What are the ingredients in Liquor Zinci Chloridi?

Zinc.
Hydrochloric Acid.
Nitric Acid.
Precipitated Zinc Carbonate.
Distilled Water.

410. How is Zinci Phosphidum prepared?

By passing vapors of phosphorus in a current of dry hydrogen over fused zinc.

IRON.

411. *What is the U. S. P. definition of Ferrum?

Metallic iron in the form of fine, bright, non-elastic wire.

412. *How is Tincture of Ferric Chloride made?

By diluting Solution of Ferric Chloride with alcohol, and allowing it to stand for three months.

413. *Why is it allowed to stand for three months?

To permit the formation of compound ethers, which are produced by the action of the free acid on the alcohol.

414. How does Ferri et Quininæ Citris Solubilis differ from Ferri et Quininæ Citras?

The soluble citrate contains ammonia water, and is soluble; the other does not, and is not soluble.

415. *How much Strychnine in Iron and Strychnine Citrate?

One per cent.

416. *Why is sugar used in the iron preparations?

To prevent oxidation.

417. *What is the difference between Liquor Ferri Subsulphatis and Liquor Ferri Tersulphatis.

The Liquor Ferri Subsulphatis contains more iron and less sulphuric acid than the Liquor Ferri Tersulphatis.

418. *Give the distinguishing test between the above solutions.

The solution of Subsulphate of Iron gives a white precipitate with sulphuric acid. The solution of the Tersulphate gives a clear solution with the same reagent.

419. *What would you dispense if a Solution of Persulphate of Iron was prescribed?

The solution of Subsulphate of Iron.

420. What form of iron is used in making the Scale Salts of Iron?

Ferric Hydrate.

SILVER.

421. *In what form is Silver usually found?
As Sulphide; usually associated with lead.

422. *Why was Silver Cyanide made official?
For the extemporaneous preparation of Hydrocyanic Acid.

423. What is the most important salt of Silver?
Silver Nitrate.

MERCURY.

424. What is the synonym for Mercury Sulphide?
Cinnabar.

425. *How many official preparations contain metallic Mercury?
Five.

426. *How many series of compounds does Mercury form?
Two. Mercurous and Mercuric.

427. State which, Corrosive Sublimate or Calomel, contains the more mercury.
Calomel.

428. *Which is the more poisonous, the Red Iodide or the Yellow Iodide of Mercury?
The Red Iodide.

429. *What is the chemical test between the Yellow and Red Oxide of Mercury?
When the yellow oxide is digested with a solution of oxalic acid, it turns white. The red oxide is not changed by the same process.

430. *What is the amount of the active ingredient in each of the following by per cent.?

Acidum Aceticum Dilutum 6
Acidum Aceticum......................36
Acidum Aceticum Glaciale............99
Acidum Hydrocyanicum Dilutum....2
Acidum Hydrochloricum............31.9
Acidum Lacticum....................75
Acidum Sulphuricum............ ...92.5
Aqua Ammoniae..... 10
Aqua Ammoniae Fortior.............28
Aqua Hydrogenii Dioxide...... 3
Aqua Creosoti.............................1
Alcohol ....By weight 91
Alcohol Absolutum ..... " " 99
Alcohol Deodoratum... " " 92.5
Alcohol Dilutum.......... " " 41
Chloroformium .... 99 to 99.4
Emplastrum Hydrargyri............30
Extractum Nucis Vomicae 15
Extractum Nucis Vomicae Fluidum
....1.5
Extractum Opii 18
Ferri et Quininae Citras......Quin. 12
Ferri et Strychninae Citras, Strych 1
Infusum Digitalis.. ....1.5
Infusum Cinchonae........................ 6
Liquor Acidi Arsenosi.....................1
Liquor Calcis....................0.17
Liquor Ferri Subsulphatis.... ...... 13.6
Liquor Ferri Tersulphatis 8
Liquor Plumbi Subacetatis.............25
Liquor Potassae 5
Liquor Potassii Arsenitis...... 1

Liquor Sodii Arsenatis......................1
Liquor Zinci Chloridi....................50
Mucilago Acaciae........................34
Oleatum Hydrargyri...................... 20
Oleatum Veratrinae........................2
Opii Pulvis......................13 to 15
Opium 9
Spiritus Ammoniae......................10
Spiritus Camphorae 10
Spiritus Chloroformi.._... 6
Spiritus Frumenti....................44 to 50
Spiritus Glonoini............................1
Spiritus Phosphori....................0.12
Syrupus Acidi Citrici....................1
Syrupus Calcis 5
Syrupus Ferri Iodidi....................10
Syrupus Scillae Compositus, Tartar
Emetic 0.2
Tinctura Aconiti....................—.35
Tinctura Carnnabis Indicae........... 15
Tinctura Capsici...................... 5
Tinctura Cinchonae 25
Tinctura Colchici Seminis.............10
Tinctura Digitalis 15
Tinctura Iodi...................... 7
Tinctura Lactucarii...................... 50
Tinctura Nucis Vomicae (Alkaloids)
.... --- 0.3
Tinctura Opii (Opium...10) Morphine
....1.3 to 1.5
Tinctura Straphanthi 5
Tinctura Veratri Viridis...............40

Botany.

1. *What is Botany?

Botany is the science which treats of the structure of plants, the functions of their parts, their classification, and the terms which are employed in their description.

2. *What is a Root?

The descending axis of a plant.

3. *What is a Rhizome?

A stem remaining wholly or partly under ground and growing mostly in a horizontal or oblique direction.

4. *What is a Tuber?

A tuber is the enlarged portion of an underground stem, possessing latent buds called eyes.

5. *What is a Bulb?

A subterranean leaf bud with fleshy leaves called scales.

6. What is a Corm?

The dilated, fleshy, tuberous-base of an annual stem.

7. *What is a Flower?

That part of a plant which contains the organs of fructification.

8. *What is a male flower?

A flower with stamens and no pistils. (Sterile.)

9. *What is a female flower?

A flower with pistils and no stamens.

10. *What are Stamens?

The male organs of flowers.

11. *What are Pistils?

The female organs of flowers.

12. *What is the Ovary of a Flower?

The part of the pistil which contains the ovules.

13. What is Pollen?

The yellow dust in the anther.

14. *What is the Stigma?

The part of the plant which receives the pollen.

15. *What is the Inflorescence of a plant?

The part of the plant which bears the flowers and fruit.

16. *What is an Ovule?

The body which, after fertilization, becomes the seed.

17. *What is a Seed?

The fully developed and ripened ovule.

18. *What is a Fruit?

The ripened ovary of a flower.

19. What are Aggregated Fruits?

Fruits that consist of a mass of simple fruits, all the product of a simple flower.

20. What are Collective Fruits?

Fruits that are the product of numerous distinct flowers growing in compact clusters.

21. What is a Drupaceous Fruit?

A stone fruit, as the peach and cherry.

22. Define Pericarp.

The pericarp is the part of the fruit that contains the seed.

23. Define Sarcocarp.

The fleshy part of a drupaceous fruit.

24. *What is a Berry?

> A succulent or pulpy fruit containing naked seeds.

25. *What are Leaves?

> Leaves are the organs of respiration of a plant.

26. What is a Leaflet?

> A separate blade of a compound leaf.

27. What is a Compound Leaf?

> A leaf composed of leaflets.

28. What is a Netted Leaf?

> A leaf in which the veins form a network.

29. What is a Deciduous Leaf?

> A leaf lasting for one season only.

30. What is a Serrate Leaf?

> A leaf with notched edges.

31. What are Stomata?

> Breathing pores. They are usually on the under side of the leaf.

32. *What is Chlorophyl?

> The green coloring matter of a leaf.

33. *What do you understand by the term Spore?

> The reproductive body in non-flowering plants.

34. What is meant by the Habitat of a plant?

> The character of the place in which the plant grows wild.

35. *What is a Parasitic Plant?.

> A plant that grows upon and derives its nourishment from another plant.

36. *What is a Biennial Plant?

> A plant which requires two years to grow and mature its fruit, growing one year and flowering and fruiting the next.

37. *Define Thallus.

A vegetative body undifferentiated into root stem or leaves.

38. *What do you understand by the term Fungi?

A general term for those flowerless plants which contain no chloro-phyl and are either parasitic or soprophytic.

39. Define Sclerotium.

A consolidated and hardened mass of hyphæ in a resting condition, as in ergot.

40. What is an Herb?

A plant in which the stem does not become woody, but dies to the ground annually after flowering.

41. What is a Shrub?

A perennial woody plant with many stems branching from near the ground, generally smaller than a tree.

Organic Drugs.

What is the Botanical name and the part used of the following?

Absinthium—The leaves and tops of Artemisia Absinthium. Nat. Ord., Compositæ. Dose, 20 gr.

Acacia—A gummy exudation from Acacia Senegal. Nat. Ord., Leguminosae.

Aconitum—The tuberous root Aconitum Napellus. Nat. Ord., Ranunculaceae. Dose, 2 gr.

Allium—The bulb of Allium Sativum. Nat. Ord., Liliaceae. Dose, 60 gr.

Aloe Barbadensis—The inspissated juice of the leaves of Aloe vera. Nat. Ord., Liliaceae. Dose, 10 gr.

Aloe Socotrina—The inspissated juice of the leaves of Aloe Perryi. Nat. Ord., Liliaceae. Dose, 20 gr.

Ammoniacum—A gum resin obtained from Dorema Ammoniacum. Nat. Ord., Umbelliferae. Dose, 30 gr.

Amygdala Amara—The seed of Prunus Amygdalus. Var., Amara. Nat. Ord., Rosaceae.

Amygdala Dulcis—The seed of Prunus Amygdalus. Var., dulcis. Nat. Ord., Rosaceae.

Amylum—The fecula of the seed of Zea Mays. Nat. Ord.. Gramineae.

Althaea—The root of Althaea officinalis. Nat. Ord., Malvaceae.

Anisum—The fruit of Pimpinella Anisum. Nat. Ord., Umbelliferae. Dose, 30 gr.

Authemis—The flower heads of Anthemis nobilis. Nat. Ord., Compositae. Dose, 2 dr.

Apocynum—The root of Apocynum cannabinum. Nat. Ord., Apocynaceae. Dose, 20 gr.

Arnicae Flores—The flower heads of Arnica Montana. Nat. Ord., Compositae. Dose, 20 gr.

Asafoetida—A gum resin from the root of Ferula foetida. Nat. Ord., Umbelliferae. Dose, 15 gr.

Asclepias—The root of Asclepias tuberosa. Nat. Ord., Asclepiadeae. Dose, 2 dr.

Aspedium—The rhizome of Dryopteris Felix-mass. Nat. Ord., Filices. Dose, 2 dr.

Aspidosperma—The bark of Aspidosperma quebracho blanco. Nat. Ord.. Apocynaceae. Dose, 30 gr.

Aurantii Amari Cortex—The rind of the fruit of Citrus Aurantium. Nat. Ord., Rutaceae.

Balsamum Peruvianum—A balsam obtained from Tuluifera Pereirae. Nat. Ord., Leguminosae. Dose, 30 m.

Balsamum Tolutanum—A balsam obtained from Tuluifera Balsamum. Nat. Ord., Leguminosea. Dose, 30 m.

Belladonnae Folia—The leaves of Atropa Belladonna. Nat. Ord., Solanaceae. Dose, 5 gr.

Belladonna Radix—The root of Atropa Belladonna. Nat. Ord., Solonaceae. Dose, 3 gr.

Benzoinum—A balsamic resin obtained from Styrax Benzoin. Nat. Ord., Styraceae.

Bryonia—The root of Bryonia alba. Nat. Ord., Cucurbitaceae. Dose, 60 gr.

Buchu—The leaves of Barosma Betulina. Nat. Ord., Rutaceae. Dose, 1 dr.

Calamus—The rhizome of Acorus Calamus. Nat. Ord., Aroideae. Dose, ad libitum.

Calendula—The fresh flowering herb of Calendula officinalis. Nat. Ord., Compositae.

Calumba—The root of Jateorrhiza palmata. Nat. Ord., Menispermaceae. Dose, 30 gr.

Cambogia—A gum resin obtained from Garcinia Hanburii. Nat. Ord., Guttiferae. Dose, 5 gr.

Camphor—A Stearopten derived from Cinnamomum Camphora. Nat. Ord., Laurineae. Dose, 10 gr.

Cannabis Indica—The flowering tops of the female plant of Cannabis sativa. Nat. Ord., Urticaceæ. Dose, 5 gr.

Capsicum—The fruit of Capsicum fastigiatum. Nat. Ord., Solanaceæ. Dose, 5 gr.

Cardamomum—The fruit of Ellattaria repens. Nat. Ord., Scitamineæ. Dose, 15 gr.

Carum—The fruit of Carum Carvi. Nat. Ord., Umbelliferæ. Dose, 30 gr.

Caryophyllus—The unexpanded flowers of Eugenia aromatica. Nat. Ord., Myrtaceæ. Dose, 30 gr.

Cascarilla—The bark of Croton Eluteria. Nat. Ord., Euphorbiaceæ. Dose, 30 gr.

Cassia Fistula—The fruit of Cassia Fistula. Nat. Ord., Leguminosae. Dose, 8 dr.

Castanea—The leaves of Castanae dentata. Nat. Ord., Cupuliferae. Dose, 2 dr.

Catechu—An extract prepared from the wood Acacia Catechu. Nat. Ord., Leguminosae. Dose, 30 gr.

Caulophyllum—The rhizome and roots of Caulophyllum thalictroides. Nat. Ord., Berberideae. Dose, 30 gr.

Cetraria—The thallus of Cetraria islandica. Nat. Ord., Lichenes.

Chelidonium—The entire plant of Chelidonium majus. Nat. Ord., Papaveraceae. Dose, 60 gr.

Chenopodium—The fruit of Chenopodium ambrosioides. Nat. Ord., Chenopodiaceae. Dose, 30 gr.

Chimaphila—The leaves of Chimaphila umbellata. Nat. Ord., Ericaceae. Dose, 2 dr.

Chirata—The entire plant of Swertia Chirata. Nat. Ord., Gentianeae. Dose, 20 gr.

Chondrus—The thalli of Chondrus crispus. Nat. Ord., Gigartineae.

Chrysarobinum—A neutral principle extracted from Goa Powder, a substance found deposited in the wood of Andira Araroba. Nat. Ord., Leguminosae. Dose, one-twelfth gr.

Cimicifugae—The rhizome and rootlets of Cimicifuga racemosa. Nat. Ord., Ranunculaceae. Dose, 30 gr.

Cinchona—The bark of Cinchona Calisaya, Cinchona officinalis, or any other species of Cinchona. Nat. Ord., Rubiaceae, yielding not less than 5 per cent. of total alkaloids and at least 2.5 per cent. of quinine. Dose, 4 dr.

Cinchona Rubra—The bark of Cinchona succirubra. Nat. Ord., Rubiaceae. Dose, 4 dr.

Cinnamomum Cassia—The bark of the shoots of undetermined species of Cinnamomum grown in China. Nat. Ord., Laurineae. Dose, 30 gr.

Cinnamomum Zeylanicum—The inner bark of the shoots of Cinnamomum Zeylanicum. Nat. Ord., Laurineae. Dose, 30 gr.

Coca—The leaves of Erythroxylon Coca. Nat. Ord., Lineae. Dose, 1 dr.

Coccus—The dried female of Coccus cacti (class insecta, order Hemiptera) Dose, ½ gr.

Colchici Radix—The corm of Colchicum autumnale. Nat. Ord., Liliaceae. Dose, 8 gr.

Colchici Semen—The seed of Colchicum autumnale. Nat. Ord., Liliaceae. Dose, 5 gr.

Colocynthis—The fruit of Citrullus Colocynthis. Nat. Ord.. Cucurbitaceae. Dose, 8 gr.

Conium — The full grown fruit of Conium maculatum. Nat. Ord., Umbelliferae. Dose, 5 gr.

Convallaria—The rhizome and roots of Convallaria majalis. Nat. Ord., Liliaceae. Dose, 20 gr.

Copaiba—The oleoresin of Copaiba Langsdorffii. Nat. Ord., Leguminosae. Dose, 1 dr.

Coriandrum—The fruit of Coriandrum Sativum. Nat. Ord.. Umbelliferae. Dose, 30 gr.

Crocus—The stigmas of Crocus sativus. Nat. Ord., Irideae. Dose, 30 gr.

Cubeba—The unripe fruit of Piper Cubeba. Nat. Ord., Piperaceae. Dose, 2 dr.

Cusso—The female inflorescence of Hagenia abyssinica. Nat. Ord., Rosaceae. Dose, 4 dr.

Cypripedium—The rhizome and rootlets of Cypripedium pubescens. Nat. Ord., Orchideae. Dose, 30 gr.

Digitalis—The leaves of Digitalis purpurea. Nat. Ord., Scrophularineae. Dose, 3 gr.

Dulcamara—The young branches of Salanum Dulcamara. Nat. Ord., Solanaceae. Dose, 2 dr.

Elastica—The prepared milk juice of various species of Hevea. Nat. Ord., Euphorbiaceae.

Elaterinum—A neutral principle obtained from Elaterium, a substance deposited by the juice of Ecballium Elaterium. Nat. Ord., Cucurbitaceae. Dose, one-sixteenth gr.

Ergota—The sclerotium of Claviceps purpurea (class Fungi) replacing the grain of rye, Secale cereale. Nat. Ord., Gramineae. Dose, 30 gr.

Eriodictyon—The leaves of Eriodictyon glutenosum. Nat. Ord., Hydrophylaceae. Dose, 30 gr.

Eucalyptus—The leaves of Eucalyptus globulus. Nat. Ord., Myrtaceae. Dose, 1 dr.

Euonymus—The bark of Euonymus atropurpureus. Nat. Ord., Celastrineae. Dose, 2 gr.

Ficus—The fleshy receptacle of Ficus Carica. Nat. Ord., Urticaceae. Dose freely.

Foeniculum—The fruit of Foeniculum Capillaceum. Nat. Ord., Umbelliferae. Dose, 2 gr.

Galla—An excrescence on Quercus Insitanica (Nat. Ord., Cupuliferae) made by the sting of the gall fly, Cynips Gallae tinctoria (class insecta; order Hymenoptera). Dose, 2 dr.

Gelsemium—The rhizome and rootlets of Gelsemium sempervirens. Nat. Ord., Loganaceae. Dose, 10 gr.

Gentiana—The root of Gentiana lutea. Nat. Ord., Gentianeae. Dose, 30 gr.

Geranium—The rhizome of Geranium maculatum. Nat. Ord., Geraniaceae, Dose, 1 dr.

Glycyrrhiza—The root of Glycyrrhiza glabra. Nat. Ord., Leguminosae. Dose freely.

Gossypii Radicis Cortex—The bark of the root of Gossypium herbaceum. Nat. Ord., Malvaceae. Dose, 1 dr.

Gossypium Purificatum—The hairs of the seed of Gossypium herbaceum, freed from impurities and deprived of fatty matter.

Granatum—The bark and root of Punica Granatum. Nat. Ord., Lythrarieae. Dose, 1 dr.

Grindelia—The leaves and flowering tops of Grindelia robusta. Nat. Ord., Compositae. Dose, 1 dr.

Guaiaci Lignum—The heart wood of Guaiacum officinale. Nat Ord., Zygophylleae. Dose, 1 dr.

Guaiaci Resina—The resin of the wood of Guaiacum officinale. Nat. Ord., Zygophylleae. Dose, 30 gr.

Guarana—A dry paste prepared from the crushed seed of Paullinia sorbilis. Nat. Ord., Sapindaceae.

Hamamelis—The leaves of Hamamelis virginia. Nat. Ord., Hamamelaceae.

Hedeoma—The leaves and tops of Hedeoma pulegioides. Nat. Ord., Labiatae.

Humulus—The strobiles of Humulus Lupulus. Nat. Ord., Urticaceae.

Hydrastis—The rhizome and rootlets of Hydrastis canadensis. Nat. Ord., Ranunculaceae.

Hyoscyamus—The leaves of Hyoscyamus niger. Nat. Ord., Solanaceae. Dose, 15 gr.

Illicium—The fruit of Illicium verum. Nat. Ord., Magnoliaceae. Dose, 30 gr.

Inula—The root of Inula helenium. Nat. Ord., Compositae. Dose, 1 dr.

Ipecacuanha—The root of Cephalis Ipecacuanha. Nat. Ord., Rubiaceae. Dose, 30 gr.

Iris—The rhizome and rootlets of Iris versicolor. Nat. Ord., Irideae. Dose, 30 gr.

Jalapa—The tuberous root of Ipomaea Jalapa. Nat. Ord., Convolvulaceae. Dose, 30 gr.

Juglans—The inner bark of the root of Juglans cinerae. Nat. Ord., Juglandaceae. Dose, 2 dr.

Kamala—The glands and hairs from the capsules of Mallotus philippinensis. Nat. Ord., Euphorbiaceae. Dose, 2 dr.

Kino—The inspissated juice Pterocarpus Marsupium. Nat. Ord., Leguminosae. Dose, 30 gr.

Krameria—The root of Krameria triandra. Nat. Ord., Polygaleae. Dose, 30 gr.

Lactucarium—The concrete milk juice of Lactuca virosa. Nat. Ord., Compositae. Dose, 20 gr.

Lappa—The root of Arctium Lappa. Nat. Ord., Compositae. Dose, 1 dr.

Leptandra—The rhizome and rootlets of Veronica virginica. Nat. Ord., Scrophularineae. Dose, 1 dr.

Limonis Cortex—The rind of the fruit of Citrus Limonum. Nat. Ord., Rutaceae.

Linum—The seed of Linum usitatissimum. Nat. Ord., Lineae.

Lobelia—The leaves and tops of Lobelia inflata. Nat. Ord., Lobeliaceae. Dose, 10 gr.

Lupulinum—The glandular powder separated from the strobiles of Humulus Lupulus. Nat. Ord., Urticaceae. Dose, 15 gr.

Lycopodium—The spores of Lycopodium clavatum. Nat. Ord., Lycopodiaceae.

Macis—The arillode of the seed of Myristica fragrans. Nat. Ord., Myristicaceae. Dose, 20 gr.

Manna—The concrete saccharine exudation of Fraxinus Ornus. Nat. Ord., Oleaceae. Dose, 1 oz.

Marrubium—The leaves and tops of Marrubium Vulgare. Nat. Ord., Labiatae. Dose, 2 dr.

Mastiche—A concrete resinous exudation from Pistacia Lentiscus. Nat. Ord., Anacardieae.

Matico—The leaves of Piper Augustifolium. Nat. Ord., Piperaceae. Dose, 2 dr.

Matricaria—The flower heads of Matricaria Chamomilla. Nat. Ord., Compositae. Dose, 2 dr.

Melissa—The leaves and tops of Melissa officinalis. Nat. Ord., Labiatae. Dose, 2 dr.

Menispermum—The rhizome and roots of menispermum canadense. Nat. Ord,, Menispermaceae. Dose, 30 gr.

Mentha Piperita—The leaves and tops of Mentha piperita. Nat. Ord., Labiatae.

Mentha Viridis—The leaves and tops of Mentha viridis. Nat. Ord., Labiatae.

Mezereum—The bark of Daphne Mezereum. Nat. Ord., Thymelaceae. Dose, 15 gr.

Myristica—The seed of Myristica fragrans. Nat. Ord., Myristicaceae. Dose, 15 gr.

Myrrha—A gum resin obtained from Commiphora Myrrha. Nat. Ord., Burseraceae. Dose, 30 gr.

Nux Vomica—The seed of Strychnos Nux-vomica. Nat. Ord., Loganiaceae. Dose, 4 gr.

5 e

Opium—The concrete milky exudation obtained by incising the unripe capsules of Papaver Somniferum. Nat. Ord., Papaveraceae. Dose, 2 gr.   .

Pareira—The root of Chondodendron tomentosum. Nat. Ord., Menispermaceae. Dose, 1 dr.

Pepo—The seed of Cucurbita Pepo. Nat. Ord., Cucurbitaceae. Dose, 3 oz.

Physostigma—The seed of Physostigma venenosum. Nat. Ord., Leguminosae. Dose, 2 gr.

Phytolaccae Radix—The root of Phytolaccae decandra. Nat. Ord., Phytolaccaceae. Dose, 30 gr.

Picro'oxinum—A neutral principle obtained from the seed of Animerta paniculata. Nat. Ord., Menispermaceae. Dose, 1-60 gr.

Pilocarpus—The leaflets of Pilocarpus selloanus. Nat. Ord., Rutaceae. Dose, 60 gr.   .

Pimenta—The fruit of Pimenta officinalis. Nat. Ord., Myrtaceae. Dose, 30 gr.

Piper—The unripe fruit of Piper nigrum. Nat. Ord., Piperaceae. Dose 20 gr.

Pix Burgundica—The prepared resinous exudation from Abies excelsa. Nat. Ord., Coniferae.

· Podophyllum—The rhizome and rootlets of Podophyllum peltatum. Nat. Ord., Berberidaceae.

Prunum—The fruit of Prunus domestica. Nat. Ord., Rosaceae.

Pulsatilla—The herb of Anemone Pulsatilla. Nat. Ord., Ranunculaceae. Dose, 5 gr.

Pyrethrum—The root of Anacyclus Pyrethrum. Nat. Ord., Compositae. Dose, 1 dr.

Quassia—The wood of Picraena excelsa. Nat. Ord., Simarubeae.

Quercus Alba—The bark of Quercus alba. Nat. Ord., Cupuliferae. Dose, 1 dr.

Quillaja—The inner bark of Quillaja Saponaria. Nat. Ord., Rosaceae. Dose, 30 gr.

Rhamnus Purshiana—The bark of Rhamnus Purshiana. Nat. Ord., Rhamnaceae. Dose, 1 dr,

Rheum—The root of Rheum officinale. Nat. Ord., Polygonaceae. Dose, 30 gr.

Rhus Glabra—The fruit of Rhus glabra. Nat. Ord., Anacardieae. Dose, 1 dr.

Rhus Toxicodendron—The leaves of Rhus radicans. Nat. Ord., Anacardieae. Dose, 5 gr.

Rosa Centifolia—The petals of Rosa centifolia. Nat. Ord., Rosaceae.

Rosa Gallica—The petals of Rosa gallica. Nat. Ord., Rosaceae.

Rubus—The bark of the root of Rubus villosus. Nat. Ord., Rosaceae.

Rubus Idaeus—The fruit of Rubus Idaeus. Nat. Ord., Rosaceae.

Rumex—The root of Rumex Crispus. Nat. Ord., Polygonaceae. Dose, 1 dr.

Sabina—The tops of Juniperus Sabina. Nat. Ord., Coniferae. Dose, 15 gr.

Saccharum—A refined sugar obtained from Saccharum officinarum, and from various species and varieties of Sorghum. Nat. Ord., Gramineae, from one or more varieties of Beta vulgaris. Nat. Ord., Chenopodiaceae.

Salvia—The leaves of salvia officinalis. Nat. Ord., Labiatae. Dose, 1 dr.

Sambucus—The flowers of Sambucus canadensis. Nat. Ord., Caprifoliaceae. Dose, 1 dr.

Sanguinaria—The rhizome of Sanguinaria canadensis. Nat. Ord., Papaveraceae. Dose, 30 gr.

Santalum Rubrum—The wood of Pterocarpus santalinus. Nat. Ord., Leguminosae.

Santonica—The unexpanded flower heads of Artemisia pauciflora. Nat. Ord., Compositae. Dose, 15 gr.

Sarsaparilla—The root of Similax officinalis. Nat. Ord., Liliaceae. Dose, 1 dr.

Sassafras—The bark of the root of Sassafras variifolium. Nat. Ord., Laurineae. Dose, 1 dr.

Sassafras Medulla—The pith of Sassafras variifolium. Nat. Ord., Laurineae.

Scammonium—A resinous exudation from the living root of Convolvulus Scammonia. Nat. Ord., Convolvulaceae. Dose, 15 gr.

Scilla—The sliced bulb of Urginea maritima. Nat. Ord., Liliaceae. Dose, 3 gr.

Scoparius—The tops of Cytissus Scoparius. Nat. Ord., Leguminosae. Dose, 1 dr.

Scutellaria—The herb of Scutellaria lateriflora. Nat. Ord., Labiatae. Dose, 2 dr.

Senega—The root of Polygala Senega. Nat. Ord., Polygonaceae. Dose, 20 gr.

Senna—The leaflets of Cassia acutifolia and Cassia angustifolia. Nat. Ord., Leguminosae. Dose, 2 dr.

Serpentaria—The rhizome and roots of Aristolochia Serpentaria. Nat. Ord., Aristolochiaceae. Dose, 30 gr.

Sinapis Alba—The seed of Brassica alba. Nat. Ord., Cruciferae. Dose, 4 dr.

Sinapis Nigra—The seed of Brassica nigra. Nat. Ord., Cruciferae. Dose, 4 dr.

Spigelia—The rhizome and rootlets of Spigelia marilandica. Nat. Ord., Loganiaceae. Dose, 2 dr.

Staphisagria—The seed of Delphinium Staphisagria. Nat. Ord., Ranunculaceae.

Stillingia—The root of Stillingia sylvatica. Nat. Ord., Euphorbiaceae. Dose, 1 dr.

Stramonii Semen—The seed of Datura Stramonium. Nat. Ord., Solanaceae. Dose, 3 gr.

Stramonii Folia—The leaves of Datura Stramonium. Nat. Ord., Solanaceae. Dose, 5 gr.

Strophanthus—The seed of Strophanthus hispidus. Nat. Ord., Apocynaceae.

Styrax—A balsam prepared from the inner bark of Liquidambar orientalis. Nat. Ord., Hamamelaceae. Dose, 20 gr.

Sumbul—The root of Ferula Sumbul. Nat. Ord., Umbellifera. Dose, 60 gr.

Tabacum—The commercial dried leaves of Nicotina Tabacum. Nat. Ord., Solanaceae. Dose, 5 gr.

Tamarindus—The preserved pulp of the fruit of Tamarindus indica. Nat. Ord., Leguminosae. Dose, 1 oz.

Tanacetum—The leaves and tops of Tanacetum vulgare. Nat. Ord., Compositae. Dose, 4 dr.

Terebinthina—A concrete oleo-resin obtained from Pinus palustris and other species of Pinus. Nat. Ord., Coniferae. Dose, 30 m.

Terebinthina Canadensis—A liquid oleo-resin obtained from Abies balsamea. Nat. Ord., Conifera. Dose, 30 m.

Thymol—A phenol occuring in the volatile oils of Thymus vulgaris and Monarda punctata. Nat. Ord., Labiatae. Dose, 2 gr.

Tragacantha—A gummy exudation from Astragalus gummifer. Nat. Ord., Leguminosae.

Triticum—The rhizome of Agropyrum repens. Nat. Ord., Gramineae. Dose, 2 dr.

Ulmus—The bark of Ulmus fulva. Nat. Ord., Urticaceae.

Valeriana—The rhizome and rootlets of Valeriana officinalis. Nat. Ord., Valerianaceae. Dose, 30 gr.

Vanilla—The fruit of Vanilla planifolia. Nat. Ord., Orchideae.

Veratrina—A mixture of Alkaloids obtained from the seed of Asagraea officinalis. Nat. Ord., Liliaceae. Dose, one-tenth gr.

Veratrum Viride—The rhizome and rootlets of Veratrum Viride. Nat. Ord., Liliaceae. Dose, 5 gr.

Viburnum Opulus—The bark of Viburnum Opulus. Nat. Ord., Caprifoliaceae. Dose, 2 dr.

Xanthoxylum—The bark of Xanthoxylum americanum. Nat. Ord., Rutaceae. Dose, 30 gr.

Zingiber—The rhizome of Zingiber officinale. Nat. Ord., Scitamineae. Dose. 15 gr.

Miscellaneous.

Questions on Materia Medica.

1. *What is Camphor? Name adulterants.

   A stearopten. Adulterated with Borneo Camphor, Paraffin, Ammonium Chloride.

2. *What official drug must be one year old before being used?

   Frangula.

3. *What two official drugs must not be used when more than a year old?

   Ergot, Pulsatilla.

4. Name two true balsams.

   Balsam of Tolu, Balsam of Peru.

5. *What two official drugs in the Nat. Ord. Scitamineae?

Cardamom, Ginger.

6. What alkaloids are found in Ipecac?

Emetine, Choline.

7. *What is the botanical name of the plant from which Oil of Rose is obtained?

Rosa Damascena.

8. Name a sudorific leaf drug, a rubefacient seed drug, and a poisonous rhizome drug.

(a) Pilocarpus.
(b) Sinapis Nigra.
(c) Gelsemium.

9. *Name two gum resins in the Nat. Ord. Umbelliferae.

Ammoniac, Asafoetida.

10. Name three drugs whose chief property is astringent.

Catechu, Kino, Galla.

11. *Name two narcotic drugs.

Opium, Belladonna.

12. *What three drugs are used solely as bitter tonics?

Gentian, Quassia, Calumba.

13. Name three drugs that are emmenagogue?

Cimicifuga, Ergot, Cotton Root Bark.

14. *What two drugs are used chiefly as anthelmintics?

Chenopodium, Santonica.

15. *What two drugs are used chiefly as a taenifuge?

Kamala, Aspidium.

16. Name two drugs that are irritant; one a leaf drug and one a bark drug.

Rhus Toxicodendron (leaf), Mezereum (bark).

17. *Name three drugs recognized as oxytocics.

Cotton Root Bark, Oil of Savin, Oil of Tansy.

18. What is Red Saunders?

The wood Pterocarpus Santalinus.

19. What is Sandal Wood?

The wood of Santalum album.

20. *What are the active ingredients in Senna, Cantharides, Cocculus Indicus?

(a) Cathartic Acid.
(b) Cantharidin.
(c) Picrotoxin.

21. What is the principal drying oil?

Linseed Oil.

22. *Name two drugs of which the unexpanded flower is the part used.

Clove, the unexpanded flower of Eugenia aromatica; and Santonica, the unexpanded flower of Artemisia panciflora.

23. What is the source of Butter of Cacao?

The seed of Theobroma Cacao.

24. *How many Cinnamons are official? Name them.

Three. Cinnamomum Cassia, Cinnamomum Saigonicum, Cinnamomum Zeylanicum.

25. What is Picrotoxin?

A neutral principle obtained from the seed of Anamerta paniculata.

26. *What is Spartine Sulphate?

The neutral sulphate of an alkaloid obtained from Scoparius.

27. What action have alkaloids on litmus paper?

Turn red litmus paper blue.

28. *Name two drugs that dilate the pupil, and two that contract it.

(a) Belladonna, Stramonium.
(b) Opium, Physostigma.

29. Name two Oleoresins, two Resins, and two Gum Resins.

(a) Copaiba, Canada Turpentine.
(b) Scammony, Mastic.
(c) Gamboge, Myrrh.

30. *What is Santonine? What preparation is made from it?

A neutral principle obtained from Santonica. Official preparation, Troche.

31. Give use and dose of Kamala; use and dose of Cusso.

(a) Taenifuge. Dose, 2 dr.
(b) Anthelmintic and Taenifuge. Dose, 6 dr.

32. What is Elaterin? Give source and dose.

A neutral principle obtained from Elaterium. Dose, 1-16 gr.

33. *What are the U. S. P. requirements of Cinchona bark?

Must yield 5 per cent. of total alkaloids, one-half of which must be quinine.

34. *Why should Wild Cherry Bark be gathered in the autumn?

It yields more hydrocyanic acid and contains more tannin.

35. *What two important alkaloids are obtained from Hyoscyamus?

Hyoscyamine, Hyoscine.

36. What are the official salts of Hyoscyamine?

Hyoscyamine Hydrobromate, Hyoscyamine Sulphate.

37. Name the official preparations of Stramonium, and state what part of the plant they are made from?

Extract of Stramonium Seed, Fluid Extract of Stramonium Seed, Tincture of Stramonium Seed. All made from the seed.

38. Name one drug in the Nat Ord. Lauriniae; one in the Nat. Ord. Umbelliferae; and one in the Nat. Ord. Guttiferae.

(a) Camphor.
(b) Conium.
(c) Gamboge.

39. What is Eucalyptol?

A neutral body obtained from the volatile oil of Eucalyptus globulus.

40. *What two drugs in the Nat. Ord. Berberideae?

Caulophyllum, Podophyllum.

41. What is the chemical name for Volatile Oil of Mustard?

Allyl iso-thiocyanate.

42. What kinds of Cinchona are used in the Tinctures of Cinchona?

The compound tincture contains the Red Cinchona. The simple tincture contains Cinchona.

43. *To what is the astringent property of Rhubarb due?

To rheo-tannic acid.

44. *How does the alkaloid Morphine differ from other alkaloids?

It is precipitated by alkalies but is soluble in excess.

45. What poison is derived from one of the official substances of animal origin?

Cantharidin.

46. *From what is Veratrine obtained? Name official preparations.

From the seed of Asagraea officinalis. Oleate of Veratrine and Ointment of Veratrine.

47. What are the official preparations of Nux Vomica? What is the alkaloidal strength of each?

Fluid Extract 1.5 and Extract 15, Tincture 0.3 made from the extract.

48. *In what different forms is Opium official?

Opium, Powdered Opium and Deodorized Opium.   •

49. Give the official names of the two Chamomiles.

Anthemis, Matricaria.

50. *How can Opium be deodorized? What principle is removed?

(a) By treating it with ether.
(b) Narcotine.

51. What are the official preparations of Colchicum (a) seed, (b) of the root?

(a) Fluid Extract of Colchicum Seed.
    Tincture of Colchicum Seed.
    Wine of Colchicum Seed.
(b) Extract of Colchicum Root.
    Fluid Extract of Colchicum Root.
    Wine of Colchicum Root.

52. What U. S. P. drug is nearly pure olein?

Expressed oil of Almond.

53. *Name two sources of Oil of Anise.

Pimpinella Ainsum. Illicium Verum.

54. Give adulterants of vanilla.

Tonka Bean, Synthetic Vanillin.

55. *State the difference between Oil of Nutmeg and Oil of Mace.

Oil of Nutmeg is a volatile oil made by distilling nutmegs. Oil of Mace is a fixed oil made by expressing nutmegs.

56. *Is Oil of Sweet Almond obtained from the bitter or sweet almond, and by what process?

From either the bitter or the sweet almond, by expression.

57. *From what and by what process is Oil of Bitter Almond obtained?

From the bitter almond by maceration with water and subsequent distillation.

58. *Name three sources of Synthetic Vanillin.

Eugenol, Coniferon, Benzoin. .

59. Name two drugs that contain Berberine.

Hydrastis, Calumba.

60. Give the U. S. P. definition of an official twig.

The young branches of Solanum Dulcamara. Nat. Ord., Solanaceae.

61. *What five drugs contain volatile or amorphous alkaloids?

Tobacco, Lobelia, Scoparius, Conium and Ergot.

62. From what is Hygrine obtained?

From the leaves of Erythroxylon Coca.

63. What part of Calocynth is used?

The fruit.

64. *What acid is made from Oil of Wintergreen?
Salicylic Acid.

65. From what part of the plant is Atropine chiefly obtained?
The root.

66. Name three official drugs that yield Sulphurated Volatile oils.
Sinapis Nigra, Asafoetida, Allium.

67. *Name two crude drugs that have been standardized?
Jalap, Opium.

68. What is the Synonym for the alkaloid in Calabar Bean?
Eserine.

69. What is the official name for Artificial Oil of Wintergreen?
Merthyl Salicylate.

70. *Give the U. S. P. definition of three drugs containing Glucosides.
Santonica, the unexpanded flower heads of Artimesia pauciflora. Nat. Ord., Compositae. The rhizome and roots of Convallaria majalis. Nat. Ord., Liliaceae. Strophanthus, the seed of Strophanthus hispidus (Nat. Ord., Apocynaceae) deprived of its long awn.

71. *What seed drug yields a drastic and vesicant fixed oil?
The seed of Croton Tiglium.

72. What fruit drug has an odor like that of mice?
Conium.

73. What is Adeps Lanae Hydrosus?

The purified fat of the wool of sheep.

74. What is Chrysarobin?

A neutral principle extracted from Goa Powder, a substance found deposited in the wood of Andira Araroba. Nat. Ord., Leguminosae.

75. What is Catechu?

An extract prepared from the wood of Acacia Catechu. Nat. Ord., Leguminosae.

76. What is Kino?

The inspissated juice of Pterocarpus Marsupium. Nat. Ord., Leguminosae.

SYNONYMS.

The Latin official names and the most common synonyms of the following are:

Absinthium	Wormwood.
Acetanilidum	Antifebrin.
Acetum Opii	Black Drop.
Aconitum	Monk's Hood.
Antipyrine	Metosin.
Acidum Carbolicum	{ Phenic Acid. Phenol.
Acidum Citricum	Acid of Lemons.
Acidum Hydrochloricum	{ Muriatic Acid. Spirit of Salt.
Acidum Nitricum	Aqua Fortis.
Acidum Nitro-Hydrochloricum	Aqua Regia.
Acidum Tannicum	{ Gallotannic Acid. Digallic Acid.
Acidum Sulphuricum	Oil of Vitriol.

Acidum Sulphuricum Aromaticum.	Elixir of Vitriol.
Acidum Oxalicum	Acid of Sugar.
Alcohol	Spirit of Wine.
Ammonii Carbonas	{ Hartshorn. { Sal Volatile.
Ammonii Chloridum	Sal Ammoniac.
Antimonii Sulphuratum	Kermes Mineral.
Antimonii et Potassi Tartras	Tartar Emetic.
Apocynum	Canadian Hemp.
Anthemis	Chamomile.
Asclepias	Pleurisy Root.
Acidum Arsenosum	Ratsbane.
Aspidium	{ Male Fern. { Felix-mass.
Belladonna	Deadly Nightshade.
Benzinum	{ Petroleum Benzin. { Petroleum Ether.
Caffeina	Theine.
Calcii Sulphas Exsiccatus	{ Dried Gypsum. { Plaster of Paris.
Calendula	Marigold.
Calx Chlorata	Bleaching Powder.
Cantharis	Spanish Flies.
Capsicum	{ Cayenne Pepper. { African Pepper. { Bird Pepper.
Carbo Animalis	Ivory Black.
Cassia Fistula	Purging Cassia.
Ceratum Resina	Basilicon Ointment.
Cetraria	Iceland Moss.
Chloral	Chloral Hydrate.
Chondrus	Irish Moss.
Cimicifuga	Black Cohosh.
Cinchona	Peruvian Bark.
Colchicum	Meadow Saffron.
Collodium Cantharidatum	Blistering Collodion.

Conium	Hemlock.
Colocynthis	Bitter Apple.
Convallaria	Lily of the Valley.
Creosotum	Oil of Smoke.
Cupri Sulphas	Blue Stone. Blue Vitriol. Roman Vitriol.
Cusso	Brayera.
Cypripedium	Lady's-slipper.
Digitalis	Fox Glove.
Dulcamara	Bittersweet.
Elastica	India Rubber.
Emplastrum Picis Cantharidatum.	Warming Plaster.
Emplastrum Plumbi	Diachylon Plaster.
Emplastrum Resina	Adhesive Plaster.
Emulsum Amygdalae	Milk of Almonds.
Ergota	Spurred Rye. Blasted Rye. Rye Smut.
Eriodictyon	Yerba Santa. Mountain Balm.
Ferri Sulphas	Vitriol of Mars. Copperas. Green Vitriol.
Ferrum Reductum	Iron by Hydrogen.
Frangula	Buckthorn.
Gelseminum	Yellow Jasmine.
Geranium	Cranesbill.
Glyceritum Vitelli	Glyconin.
Glyceritum Amylum	Starch Jelly.
Glycyrrhiza	Licorice Root. Sweet Root.
Gossypium Purificatum	Absorbent Cotton.
Haematoxylon	Logwood.
Hamamelis	Witch Hazel.
Hedeoma	Pennyroyal.

Hydrargyri Chloridum Mite	Mild Chloride of Mercury. Sub-Chloride of Mercury. Proto Chloride of Mercury.
Hydrargyri Chloridum Corrosivum	Corrosive Sublimate. Per-Chloride of Mercury. Corrosive Chloride of Murcury. Bi-Chloride of Mercury.
Hydrargyri Iodidum Flavum..........	Protoiodide of Mercury. Yellow (or Green) Iodide of Mercury.
Hydrargyri Iodidum Rubrum..........	Biniodide of Mercury. Red Iodide of Mercury.
Hydrargyri Oxidum Rubrum..........	Red Precipitate.
Hydrargyri Subsulphus Flavus.......	Queen's Yellow. Turpeth Mineral.
Hydrargyrum	Quicksilver.
Hydrargyrum Ammoniatum..........	White Precipitate.
Hydrastis........................	Yellow Root. Yellow Puccoon. Golden Seal.
Hydrargyrum Cum Creta.............	Gray Powder.
Ichthyocolla	Fish Glue.
Illicium..........................	Star Anise.
Infusum Senna Compositum..........	Black Draught.
Iris	Blue Flag.
Juglans..........................	Butternut.
Kamala...........................	Rottlera.
Krameria	Rhatany.
Lappa	Burdock.
Leptandra	Culver's Root.
Linimentum Ammonia...............	Volatile Liniment.
Linimentum Calcis	Carron Oil.

Linimentum Saponis Mollis............ Tincture of Green Soap.

Liquor Ammonii Acetatis...... .... Spirit of Mendererus.

Liquor Arseni et Hydrargyri Iodidi Donovan's Solution.

Liquor Ferri et Ammonii Acetatis .. Basham's Mixture.

Liquor Ferri Subsulphatis................. Monsel's Solution.

Liquor Iodi Compositus .... Lugol's Solution.

Liquor Plumbi Subacetatis   Goulard's Extract.

Liquor Potassii Arsenitis..................... Fowler's Solution.

Liquor Sodae Chlorata................. Labarraque's Solution.

Liquor Zinci Chloride................ Burnett's Disinfecting Fluid.

Lobelia................. .... Indian Tobacco.

Lycopodium ...., ...··· { Club Moss. } Vegetable Sulphur.

Magnesia............... .... { Light Magnesia. } Calcined Magnesia.

Magnesii Sulphas............ .... { Bitter Salts. } Epsom Salts.

Marrubium .... Horehound.

Massa Capaibae.... ....,..................... Solidified Capaiba.

Massa Ferri Carbonatis................... Vallet's Mass.

Massa Hydrargyri........................ ····· { Blue Pill. } Blue Mass.

Matricaria................................. German Chamomile.

Menispermum........................... { Yellow Parilla. } Canadian Moonseed.

Methyl Salicylas..................... Artificial Oil of Winter-green.

Mistura Ferri Composita .... Griffith's Mixture.

Mistura Glycyrrhiza Composita........ Brown Mixture.

Naphtol................................ Beta Naphtol.

Nux Vomica .... ··········· { Dog Button. } Quaker Button.

Oleum Myrciae................................. Oil of Bay.

Olibanum............................. Frankincense.

6 f

Opium	Theibacum.
Physostigma	Calabar Bean.
Phytolaccae Radix	Poke Root.
Pilocarpus	Jaborandi.
Pilulae Antimonii Compositae	Plummer's Pills.
Pimenta	Allspice.
Podophyllum	{ May Apple. { Mandrake.
Potassii et Sodii Tartras	Rochelle Salts.
Potassi Nitras	Saltpetre.
Pulvis Antimonialis	James' Powder.
Pulvis Effervescens Compositus	Seidlitz Powder.
Pulvis Jalapae Compositus	Pulvis Purgans.
Pyrogallol	Pyrogallic Acid.
Resina	Colophony.
Rhus Toxicodendron	{ Poison Ivy. { Poison Oak.
Rumex	Yellow Dock.
Salol	Phenyl Salicylate.
Sambucus	Elder.
Sanguinaria	Blood Root.
Santonica	Levant Wormseed.
Sapo Mollis	Green Soap.
Scilla	Sea Onion.
Scaparius	Broom.
Scutellaria	Skull Cap.
Sevum	Mutton Suet.
Soda	{ Caustic Soda. { Sodium Hydrate.
Sodii Boras	Borax.
Sodii Bicarbonas	Baking Soda.
Sodii Carbonas	{ Sal Soda. { Washing Soda.
Sodii Sulphas	{ Glauber Salts. { Horse Salts.

Spigelia....	Pink Root.
Spiritus Aetheris Compositus	{ Golden Tincture. Hoffman's Anodyne.
Spiritus Glonoini	Spirit of Nitroglycerin.
Spiritus Myrciae.................... ..	Bay Rum.
Staphisagria...............	Stavesacre.
Stillingia...............	{ Queen's Root. Queen's Delight.
Stramonii Semen	Jimsen Seed.
Syrupus Scillae Compositus............ ..	Cox's Hive Syrup.
Taraxicum.................. ..	Dandelion.
Terebinthina Canadensis..................	{ Canada Balsam. Balsam of Fir.
Tinctura Benzoini Composita............	Turlington's Balsam.
Tinctura Cinchonae Compositae.....	Haxham's Tincture of Bark.
Tinctura Lobeliae..................	Tincture of Indian Tobacco.
Tinctura Opii.....................	{ Tinctura Thebaica. Laudanum.
Tinctura Strophanthi............	Tincture of Indian Arrow Poison.
Triticum..................	Couch Grass.
Ulmus	{ Slipery Elm. Red Elm.
Unguentum Hydrargyri	Blue Ointment.
Unguentum Hydrargyri Nitratis......	Citrine Ointment.
Uva Ursi................	Bearberry.
Viburnum Opulus.................	Cramp Bark.
Viburnum Prunifolium	Black Haw.
Vinum Opii..................	Sydenham's Laudanum.
Xanthoxylum.................	Prickly Ash.
Zinci Oxidi..	Philosopher's Wool.
Zinci Sulphas..................	White Vitriol.

THERAPEUTICAL CLASSIFICATION OF MEDICINES.

1. *What is an Anti-emetic?

A medicine that stops vomiting.

2. *What are Anaesthetics?

Drugs that produce temporary loss or impairment of feeling.

3. *What is an Anodyne?

A medicine that relieves pain.

4. *What are Anthelmintics?

Drugs that expel worms.

5. What are Antiperiodics?

Medicines that arrest morbid periodical movements.

6. What is an Aphrodisiac?

A medicine that stimulates venereal desire.

7. *What is an Antiseptic?

Any substance that prevents or checks putrefaction.

8. What is an Astringent?

A medicine that contracts the tissues of the body and prevents excessive discharges.

9. *What is a Carminative?

A medicine that expels air from the bowels.

10. *What is a Cathartic?

A drug that causes evacuation of the bowels.

11. *What is a Cholagogue?

A medicine that increases the flow of bile.

12. *What is a Demulcent?

A substance that lubricates the surface to which applied and prevents the contact of irritating substances.

13. What is a Diaphoretic?

A drug that produces perspiration.

14. What is a Drastic?

A powerful cathartic.

15. What is a Diuretic?

A medicine that acts on the kidneys and increases the discharge of urine.

16. What is an Epispastic?

A drug that produces blisters when applied to the skin.

17. What is an Expectorant?

A medicine that facilitates expectoration.

18. *What is a Hepatic?

A drug that acts on the liver.

19. *What is a Hydrogogue?

A medicine that produces watery evacuations and is believed to expel serum.

20. *What is a Lithonthriptic?

A medicine that counteracts the formation of calculi in the urinary organs.

21. *What are Narcotics?

Drugs that cause stupefaction and in large doses are poisonous.

22. What is a Nervine?

A medicine that acts on the nervous system and allays nervous excitement.

23. *What is an Oxytocic?

A drug that causes contraction of the uterus.

24. What is a Purgative?

A medicine that physics more powerfully than a cathartic.

25. *What is a Rubefacient?

A drug that produces redness of the skin.

26. What is a Resolvent?

A medicine that allays inflammation and disperses morbid swellings.

27. What is a Refrigerant?

A medicine that depresses abnormal temperature of the body.

28. What is a Sialagogue?

A medicine that increases the flow of saliva.

29. What is a Stimulant?

A drug that temporarily increases the vital forces.

30. *What is a Styptic?

Any substance that will stop the flow of blood.

31. *What is a Sudorific?

A medicine that causes sweating.

32. *What is a Tonic?

A medicine that stimulates the nutritive processes.

33. What is a Vesicant?

A medicine that produces blisters when applied to the skin.

34. *What is a Vulnerary?

A medicine that is healing to wounds.

POSOLOGY.

1. *What is Posology?

The science of Dosage.

2. *What do you understand by the dose of a medicine?

The proper quantity to be administered at one time to produce medicinal action.

3. What is the maximum dose?

The largest dose that can be taken with safety.

4. *What is the rule for apportioning doses for children?

Add 12 to the age, divide this sum by the age, divide the maximum adult dose by this quotient, the last quotient will be the maximum dose for a child of the age taken.   Ex.—Age 12 years plus 12=24. 24 divided by 12, the age=2. 60 gr., maximum dose for an adult, divided by 2=30 gr., dose for a child 12 years of age.

5. To what extent should the Pharmacist be familiar with doses?

He should know the maximum dose of all poisonous drugs so that he may be able to detect poisonous doses in prescriptions.

6. We give below a list of the most active remedies, with the maximum dose of each.

Acetanilidum ....10 gr.
Acidum Arsenosum..$\frac{1}{16}$ gr.
Acidum Carbolicum..3 gr.
Acidum Chromicum.. ¼ gr.
Acidum Gallicum ....30 gr.
Acidum Tannicum...... ....10 gr.
Acidum Hydrochloricum............................. ......10 m.
Acidum Hydrocyanicum Dilutum...........................3 m.
Acidum Phosphoricum ....7 m.
Acidum Sulphuricum Aromaticum .... 10 m.
Acidum Sulphurosum............. ....1 dr.
Aconitum ....2 gr.

Aconitine .... $\frac{1}{350}$ gr.
Aether .... 60 m.
Aloe Purificata .... 10 gr.
Aloinum .... 2 gr.
Alumen Exsiccatum .... 30 gr.
Alumini Hydras .... 10 gr.
Ammonii Carbonas .... 15 gr.
Ammonii Iodidum .... 10 gr.
Amyl Nitras .... (By inhalation) 2 to 4 m.
Antimonii et Potassi Tartras .... 2 gr.
Antimonii Oxidum .... 3 gr.
Apomorphinae Hydrochloras .... $\frac{1}{8}$ gr.
Argenti Cyanidum .... $\frac{1}{20}$ gr.
Argenti Nitras .... $\frac{1}{2}$ gr.
Arseni Iodidum .... $\frac{1}{8}$ gr.
Atropinae Sulphas .... $\frac{1}{64}$ gr.
Aurii et Sodii Chloridum .... $\frac{1}{4}$ gr.
Belladonnae Radix .... 3 gr.
Bismuthi Citras .... 5 gr.
Bismuthi Subnitras .... 60 gr.
Caffeina Citrata .... 5 gr.
Calcii Hypophosphis .... 30 gr.
Calx Sulphurata .... 1 gr.
Calx Chlorata .... 6 gr.
Cannabis Indica .... 5 gr.
Cantharis .... 2 gr.
Cereii Oxalas .... 10 gr.
Chenopodium .... 30 gr.
Chloral .... 45 gr.
Chrysarobinum .... $\frac{1}{12}$ gr.
Coccus .... $\frac{1}{2}$ gr.
Colchici Semen .... 5 gr.
Conium .... 5 gr.
Creosotum .... 3 m.

Digitalis ....3 gr.

Elaterinum ....$\frac{1}{16}$ gr.

Ergota ....30 gr.

Extractum Aconiti ....¼ gr.

Extractum Aconiti Fluidum ....1 m.

Extractum Belladonnae Foliorum Acoholicum ....¾ gr.

Extractum Cannabis Indica ....1 gr.

Extractum Capsici Fluidum ....2 m.

Extractum Cimicifugae ....5 gr.

Extractum Colchici Radicis Fluidum ....5 m.

Extractum Colchici Radicis ....3 gr.

Extractum Colocynthidis ....2 gr.

Extractum Colocynthidis Comp. ....25 gr.

Extractum Conii ....2 gr.

Extractum Conii Fluidum ....5 m.

Extractum Digitalis ....1 gr.

Extractum Digitalis Fluidum ....2 m.

Extractum Ergota ....15 gr.

Extractum Gelsemii Fluidum ....3 m.

Extractum Hyoscyami ....3 gr.

Extractum Jalapae ....10 gr.

Extractum Lobeliae Fluidum ....5 m.

Extractum Nucis Vomicae ....1 gr.

Extractum Nucis Vomicae Fluidum ....4 m.

Extractum Opii ....1 gr.

Extractum Physostigmatis ....½ gr.

Extractum Podophylli ....5 gr.

Extractum Sabinae Fluidum ....15 m.

Extractum Sanguinariae Fluidum ....5 m.

Extractum Scillae Fluidum ....5 m.

Extractum Stramonii Seminis ....½ gr.

Extractum Veratri Viridis Fluidum ....3 m.

Fel Bovis Purificatum ....10 gr.

Ferri Chloridum ....3 gr.

Ferri et Strychninae Citras..................................5 gr.

Ferri Lactas...5 gr.

Ferri Oxidum Hydratum...........................4 dr.

Ferri Phosphas Solubilis..........................10 gr.

Ferri Pyrophosphas Solubilis.....................5 gr.

Ferri Valerianas.............................2 gr.

Ferrum Reductum..............................5 gr.

Hydrargyri Chloridum Corrosivum...............⅛ gr.

Hydrargyri Chloridum Mite....................15 gr.

Hydrargyri Cyanidum.........................⅛ gr.

Hydrargyri Subsulphas Flavus................2 gr.

Hyoscinae Hydrobromas...................$\frac{1}{100}$ gr.

Hyoscyaminae Sulphas....................$\frac{1}{64}$ gr.

Iodoformum.............................3 gr.

Iodum...................................1 gr.

Lactucarium............................10 gr.

Liquor Acidi Arsenosi....................10 m.

Liquor Arseni et Hydrargyri Iodidi.........10 m.

Liquor Ferri Subsulphatis................10 m.

Liquor Iodi Compositus..................10 m.

Liquor Potassii Arsenitis................10 m.

Menthol...............................5 gr.

Morphinae Sulphas......................¼ gr.

Naphtol...............................15 gr.

Oleoresina Capsici.....................1 m.

Oleorsina Aspidii......................1 dr.

Oleorsina Zingiberis...*...............2 m.

Oleum Amygdale Amarae.................1 m.

Oleum Phosphoratum...................5 m.

Oleum Sabina........................5 m.

Oleum Sinapis Volatile...............¼ m.

Oleum Tiglii.........................2 m.

Opium...............................2 gr.

Opium Deodoratum...................2 gr.

Paraldehydum .... ½ dr.

Phosphorus .... $\frac{1}{40}$ gr.

Physostigma .... 2 gr.

Physostigminae Salicylas .... $\frac{1}{30}$ gr.

Physostigminae Sulphas.... . ... $\frac{1}{60}$ gr.

Pilulae Phosphori 2

Plumbi Acetas .... 3 gr.

Plumbi Iodidum .... 1 gr.

Potassii Bichromas .... 1 gr.

Potassii Cyanidum .... $\frac{1}{5}$ gr.

Potassii Iodidum .... 60 gr.

Potassii Permanganas .... 3 gr.

Pulsatilla .... 5 gr.

Pulvis Antimonialis .... 10 gr.

Pulvis Morphinae Compositus .... 15 gr.

Quininae Sulphas .... 20 gr.

Quininae Valerianas .... 8 gr.

Resina Podophylli .... 2 gr.

Resorcinum .... 5 gr.

Rhus Toxicodendron .... 5 gr.

Sabina .... 15 gr.

Salol .... 15 gr.

Santonica .... 15 gr.

Santoninum .... 3 gr.

Scilla .... 3 gr.

Sinapis Alba .... 4 dr.

Sodii Arsenas .... ⅛ gr.

Sodii Boras .... 30 gr.

Sodii Phosphas .... 8 dr.

Sodii Sulphocarbolas .... 20 gr.

Sparteinae Sulphas .... 1 gr.

Spiritus Aetheris Nitrosi .... 2 dr.

Spiritus Glonoini .... 1 m.

Stramonii Semen .... 3 gr.

Sulphuris Iodidum .... 4 gr.

Strychninae Sulphas .... $\frac{1}{20}$ gr.

Syrupus Ferri Iodidi ....30 m.

Terebenum .... 10 m.

Terpini Hydras ...._5 gr.

Thymol ....2 gr.

Tinctura Aconiti.... ....___3 m.

Tinctura Cantharidis........._ ....10 m..

Tinctura Digitalis..___20 m.

Tinctura Ferri Chloridi ....30 m.

Tinctura Gelsemii.. ....15 m.

Tinctura Iodi.. ....__6 m.

Tinctura Nucis Vomicae...15 m.

Tinctura Opii.. ... . 15 m.

Tinctura Opii Camphorata.................................... ....4 dr.

Tinctura Physostigmatis ....10 m.

Tinctura Scillae.._.. ....20 m.

Tinctura Stramonii Seminis..10 m.

Tinctura Strophanthi_... ....10 m.

Tinctura Veratri Viridis.. ....5 m.

Trituratio Elaterina..----- ½ gr.

Veratrina...... ....$\frac{1}{10}$ gr.

Vinum Colchici Radicis.................... ....20 m.

Vinum Colchici Seminis...................... ....60 m.

Vinum Opii ....15 m.

Zinci Sulphas........... ....As Emetic, 10 to 60 gr.

Zinci Phosphidum ....¼ gr.

TOXICOLOGY.

1. *What is Toxicology?

     The science of poisons.

2. *What is a Poison?

Any agent capable of producing a morbid or dangerous effect upon anything endowed with life.

3. *Into what classes are Poisons divided?

Irritants, narcotics, and narcotic irritants.

4. *What are Irritant Poisons?

Poisons that produce irritation and inflammation in the stomach.

5. What are Narcotic Poisons?

Poisons which affect the brain and spinal cord, and produce insensibility.

6. What are Narcotic Irritants?

Substances which have the action of both the irritant and the narcotic poisons.

7. *What are the prominent symptoms of Aconite poisoning?

A tingling sensation in the lips, tongue and tips of the fingers, followed by vomiting, dryness and constriction of the throat, with irregular action of the heart.

8. *What are the most prominent symptoms of poisoning by Arsenic?

Nausea and faintness; burning pain in the stomach; persistent vomiting of matter, sometimes brown or gray, or streaked with blood.

9. *What are the most prominent symptoms of Belladonna poisoning?

Drowsiness, great thirst, dryness of the throat, widely dilated pupils, strong pulse and loss of speech.

10. *What are the prominent symptoms of Carbolic Acid poisoning?

The surfaces which have been in contact with the poison are whitened and hardened; a burning pain from the mouth to the stomach; lowering of the pulse and temperature, contraction of the pupils.

11. *What are the prominent symptoms of Chloral poisoning?

Deep sleep, accelerated pulse, widely dilated pupils, deep, irregular respiration. Later, the pupils contract, circulation and respiration fail.

12. What are the prominent symptoms of poisoning by Copper Salts?

The vomited matter is green.

13. What are the prominent symptoms of poisoning by Digitalis?

Nausea, vomiting, slowness of the pulse, a sense of oppression in the chest, coldness of the extremities.

14. *What are the symptoms of poisoning by Hydro-cyanic Acid?

Immediate constriction of the throat, a sense of pressure in the head; tetanic convulsions, loss of consciousness.

15. *What are the prominent symptoms of poisoning by the Mineral Acids.

Acute, burning pain extending from the throat to the stomach, vomiting of dark, tarry and highly acid material.

16. *What are the prominent symptoms of poisoning by the Caustic Alkalies?

Soapy taste, burning pain from the throat to the stomach, vomiting of alkaline substances.

17. *What are the prominent symptoms of Phosphorus poisoning?

Eructations of gas having the taste of phosphorus; the mouth when observed in the dark is frequently faintly luminous; the vomited matter also is frequently luminous.

ANTIDOTES.

1. *What is an Antidote?

   Anything used to counteract the effects of a poison.

2. *How would you antidote Aconite poisoning?

   Give emetics, stimulants external and internal, external heat; keep patient flat on back.

3. *What would you give to antidote an overdose of Arsenic?

   Ferri Oxidum Hydratum, Ferri Oxidum Hydratum cum Magnesia.

4. *What is a good antidote to Carbolic Acid?

   Emetics, or stomach pump (used with great care), albuminous substances, syrup of lime and stimulants.

5. *How would you antidote Chloroform?

   Fresh air, artificial respiration, brandy and ammonia, hypodermic injections of tincture of digitalis and atropine.

6. *What is the antidote for poisoning by Belladonna?

   Emetics, physostigma or pilocarpine, cold to heat, nitroglycerin.

7. *How would you antidote Corrosive Sublimate?

   Give albumen, white of egg, equal parts of lime water and milk, followed by emetics.

8. What is the antidote for Croton Oil?

   Give emetics, wash out the stomach with mucilaginous fluids containing opium.

9. What is the antidote for Salts of Copper?

   Yellow prussiate of potash, reduced iron or soap.

10. How would you antidote Conium?

    With emetics, followed by stimulants internal and external.

11. *What is a good antidote for Cantharides?

Emetics, emollient drinks, opiates by mouth and rectum, large draughts of water to flush the kidneys.

12. How would you antidote Digitalis?

Give evacuants, stimulants internal and external, tincture of aconite.

13. What is the antidote for Elaterin?

Demulcent drinks, enemata of opium and external heat.

14. *What is the antidote for Chlorine Water?

Albumen, white of eggs, milk, flour.

15. *How would you antidote Mineral Acids?

With chalk, magnesia or any other mild alkali, emollient drinks and fixed oils.

16. *What is the chemical antidote to Salts of Silver?

Sodium chloride, forms insoluble silver chloride.

17. *How would you antidote Hydrocyanic Acid or a Cyanide?

Fresh air, artificial respiration, cold applications to the head and spine, cobaltous nitrate.

18. What is the specific antidote to Iodine?

Starch, also emetics, demulcent drinks, opium, and external heat.

19. *What is the antidote to Acute Lead poisoning?

Magnesium sulphate, followed by emetics, also opium and milk.

20. *What is the antidote to Strychnine or Nux Vomica?

Chloral, chloroform, potassium bromide, tincture of cannabis indica.

21. *How would you antidote Opium?

Emetic or stomach pump, stimulants external and internal, cold affusions, perambulatory treatment.

22. What is the antidote to Oxalic Acid?

Lime in any form. Syrup of Lime best.

23. What is the antidote to Phosphorus?

Sulphate of copper in emetic doses as a chemical antidote. Oil of turpentine has been used with good results.
Give no oily or fatty matter.

24. *How would you antidote the Caustic Alkalies?

With dilute acetic acid, citric acid, lemon juice, fixed oils and demulcents.

25. How would you antidote poisoning from inhalation of the Vapor of Ammonia?

By inhalation of the vapor of hydrochloric acid.

26. *What is the antidote to Tobacco poisoning?

Emetics, stimulants external and internal. Nux vomica.

27. *How would you antidote poisoning by Zinc Salts?

Give sodium carbonate, emetics and warm demulcent drinks.

28. In all ordinary cases of poisoning how would you proceed?

Administer a prompt emetic and send for a physician.

INCOMPATIBILITY.

1. *What is Incompatibility?

It may be defined as a term used to express the effects produced in pharmaceutical preparations by chemical decomposition or physical dissociation.

2. *Name three kinds of Incompatability?

(a) Chemical.
(b) Physical.
(c) Therapeutical.

7g

3. *What is Chemical Incompatibility?

A form of incompatability which invariably results in the decomposition of one or more of the ingredients entering into the preparation or prescription.

4. *What is Physical Incompatibility?

It is sometimes known as pharmaceutical incompatability—a condition which usually arises from the admixture of pharmaceutical preparations which result in the physical dissociation of one or more of the constituents.

5. *How does Physical Incompatibility differ from Chemical Incompatibility?

It differs from chemical incompatability in the absence of chemical action.

6. What is Therapeutical Incompatibility?

It is a condition which arises from the combination of remedies which are mutually opposed to one another in therapeutical effect.

7. Is Therapeutical Incompatibility of much interest to the pharmacist?

No. The fault lies wholly with physician.

8. *Which form of Incompatibility may be intentional on the part of the prescriber?

Chemical incompatibility is very often intentional, as in the combination of lead acetate and zinc sulphate in the same solution, the insoluble lead sulphate which is formed is the important ingredient in the preparation.

9. *What form of Incompatibility is most dangerous, and why?

Chemical. Because new, and very often poisonous, compounds are formed when chemicals react on one another.

10. *The following list of Incompatibilities should be thoroughly understood so that when met with in practice they may be recognized at once:

1. Decomposition is almost sure to take place when **strong acids** are mixed with salts.

2. Alkalies should never be mixed with salts of the metals.

3. Alkaloids should not be dispensed with alkalies.

4. Glucosides are decomposed by strong acids.

5. Alcoholic tinctures and fluid extracts are incompatible with aqueous liquids.

6. All drugs that contain tannin form inky compounds with the salts of iron.

7. The iodides are incompatible with acids.

8. Strong mineral acids decompose alcohols and form ethers.

9. Never combine free acids with carbonates or hydrates.

10. Tannin forms a precipitate in solutions that contain albumen or gelatine.

11. Vegetable infusions are generally incompatible with metallic salts.

12. Silver nitrate or oxide forms an explosive compound with ammonia.

13. Tannic acid, iodine and the soluble iodides are incompatible with alkaloids.

14. Potassium iodide and potassium chlorate form a poisonous compound, when mixed.

15. Spirit of nitrous ether is incompatible with sodium salicylate. The mixture becomes dark and develops the odor of oil of wintergreen.

16. Sodium salicylate is incompatible with quinine.

17. Potassium iodide and syrup of ferrous iodide give a precipitate of ferrous carbonate.

18. Sulphates are incompatible with lead salts; they form the insoluble lead sulphate.

19. Syrup of lactucarium is decomposed by **alkalies**.

20. The hypophosphites are incompatible with the salts of silver or mercury.

21. Potassium chlorate or permanganate will explode if triturated with tannin, sugar, sulphur, sulphides, glycerin, alcohol, tinctures or ether.

22. Almond emulsion is separated by alcoholic liquids.

23. Spirits of nitrous ether is incompatible with all drugs containing tannin.

24. Acids precipitate the sweet principle of glycyrrhiza and eriodictyon.

25. Collodion is coagulated by carbolic acid.

26. Ammoniated tincture of guaiac is incompatible with all preparations that contain salts of mercury or alkaloids.

27. Glycerin, borax and carbonates will explode if mixed.

28. All liquid preparations of opium are incompatible with lead salts; they precipitate meconate of lead.

29. All silver salts explode when triturated with organic matter.

30. Antipyrine should be dispensed alone or in simple syrup, as it is incompatible with almost everything.

31. Chloral should not be mixed with alkaline carbonates or hydrates. They form chloroform when mixed.

32. Mucilage of acacia is precipitated by solution of lead subacetate or by alcohol.

33. Never dispense a prescription that contains free nitric acid and free glycerin. They will form nitroglycerin, which is highly explosive.

34. Uva ursa is incompatible with spirits of nitrous ether.

35. Pepsin should be dispensed with acids. It will be thrown out of solution by alkalies.

36. Pancreatin is rendered inert by contact with acids.

37. Volatile oils are incompatible with aqueous liquids in quantities exceeding one drop to the fluid ounce.
38. Fixed oils and copaiba with aqueous liquids.
39. Bromides precipitate alkaloids, but the change may be prevented by the addition of a few drops of hydrochloric acid.
40. Iodine is incompatible with chloral, starch, alkalies and metallic salts.
41. Lead acetate is incompatible with hydrochloric acid, sulphuric acid and sulphates, carbonates, iodine, potassium iodide.
42. Corrosive sublimate will be decomposed, when in solution, by the addition of potassium iodide, carbonates or tannin.
43. Calomel should not be mixed with acids, acid salts, carbonates, iodine, potassium iodide.
44. Potassium iodide will be decomposed, when in solution, by the addition of lead and mercury salts, silver nitrate and chlorine water.
45. Potassium bromide must not be mixed with acids, chlorine water or the compounds of mercury.
46. Silver nitrate is incompatible with acids, acetic, hydrochloric, hydrocyanic, sulphuric; and their salts, iodine potassium iodide and potassium bromide.
47. Chlorates, nitrates and hypophosphites explode when triturated with organic substances.
48. Chromic acid explodes almost instantly with glycerin.

PRESCRIPTIONS.

1. *What is a Prescription?

A prescription may be defined as the formula which a physician writes specifying the medicinal substances he intends to be administered to a patient.

2. *What language is used in writing prescriptions and why?

> The Latin language.
> (a) Because it is the language of science.
> (b) The Latin names of drugs are nearly the same in all countries.
> (c) It is frequently advisable to withhold from the patient the names and properties of the medicines that are to be administered.

3. *Into how many parts may a prescription be divided for the purpose of study? Name them.

> Six.
> (a) The superscription.
> (b) The name of the patient.
> (c) The inscription.
> (d) The subscription.
> (e) The signa.
> (f) The name of the physician.

4. *What is the Superscription?

> This invariably consists of the symbol, $\mathbb{R}$, which is an abbreviation of of the word recipe, "take."

5. *What is the Inscription?

> The part of the prescription that contains the names and quantities of the ingredients.

6. *What is the Subscription?

> The directions to the compounder.

7. *What is the Signa?

> The directions for the patient.

8. *If you were called upon to fill a prescription, how would you proceed?

> (a) Read it carefully.
> (b) Notice bad abbreviations.
> (c) Omissions of amounts.
> (d) Transposition of amounts.
> (e) Estimation of doses.

(f) Incompatibility.
(g) Chemical Incompatibility.
(h) Intentional Incompatibility.
(i) Pharmaceutical Incompatibility.
(j) Therapeutical Incompatibility.

9. *When would you filter a prescription?

When we know that the precipitate is inert and when so ordered by the physician.

10. *How would you change the ending of nouns in the nominative case to the genitive in writing prescriptions?

Nouns ending in *a*	change to *ae*.
Nouns ending in *um* or *us*	change to *i*.
Nouns ending in *is*	change to *itis*.
Nouns ending in *as*	change to *atis*.
Nouns ending in *x*	change to *cis*.
Nouns ending in *o*	change to *inis*.
Nouns ending in *al, ol,* or *or* by adding *is*.	

11. State what, if anything, is wrong with the following Prescription:

R Chloralis .... gr. lx.
  Sodii Bicarbonatis .... gr. xc.
  Aqua Menth. Pip .... q. s. f℥iv.

Note.—The action of sodium bicarbonate on the chloral will form chloroform.

12. Would you fill this Prescription or not, and why?

R Sodii Salicylatis .... gr. xc.
  Spiriti Aetheris Nitrosi .... f℥iij.
  Quininae Sulphatis .... gr. xxx.
  Alcoholis .... f℥iv.
  Aquae Destillata .... q. s. f℥iij.

Note.—When sodium salicylate and spirits of nitrous ether are mixed, the solution turns very dark and develops the odor of oil of wintergreen. The alkaline sodium salicylate will precipitate the alkaloid quinine. The prescription should not be dispensed unless the physician can be notified of it immediately.

13. How would you dispense this in Powders?

R Chloralis...gr. lx.
Camphorae.....................................gr. lxxx.
Cocainae Hydrochloratis.....................gr. v.

Note.—Use starch to absorb the moisture, otherwise it will liquify.

14. What is wrong with the following Prescription?

R Potassii Iodidi ....gr. xl.
Acidi Nitrici.............................. ....gtt. x.
Syrupi.....................................q. s. fℨi.

Note.—The acid will liberate free iodine from the potassium iodide, which will act as an irritant poison.

15. What is the Incompatibility in the following Prescription?

R Morphinae Sulphatis................................gr. ij.
Acidi Tannici............................ gr. xxx.
Cocainae Muriatis................................gr. iij.
Aquae Destillata........................q. s. fℨij.

Note.—The tannic acid will precipitate the alkaloids.

16. What is wrong with the following Prescription?

R Hydrargyri Bichloridi.............................gr. ij.
Tincturae Guaiaci Ammoniati..............fℨiij.
Aquae...............................q. s. fℨiv.

Note.—The ammonia water will precipitate the mercury as ammoniated mercury.

17. How would you fill this prescription?

R Tincturae Ferri Chloridi..................f3iv.
Spiriti Aetheris Nitrosi ....f3ij.
Mucilagines Acaciae ....f3i.
Syrupi..................................ad. f3vi.
Misce.

Note.—Dilute the alcoholic liquids and the mucilage with syrup, and mix the whole. This will prevent the precipitation of the acacia.

18. What, if anything, is wrong with this Prescription?

R Potassii Iodidi:..................gr. xx.
Syrupi Ferri Iodidi.................f3vi.
Aquae Camphorae..............q. s. f3iv.
Misce. Fiat solutio.

Note.—This will precipitate ferrous carbonate, owing to the presence of potassium carbonate, which is combined with the potassium iodide when it is crystallized from an alkaline solution and exposed to the air.

19. Criticize the following Prescription:

R Plumbi Acetatis ....gr. xv.
Tincturae Opii ....f3iij.
Aquae..................q. s. f3vj

Note.—Precipitates meconate of lead.

20. What is wrong with the following Prescription?

R Pepsini ....gr. lx.
Sodii Boratis..................gr. xc.
Tinctura Nucis Vomicae..................f3j.
Aquae Destillata.................. q. s. f3iv.

Note.—The alkali throws the pepsin out of solution and precipitates the alkaloids in the nux vomica.

21. Criticize the following Prescription

R Hydrargyri Bichloridi............ ....gr. j.
Potassi Iodidi...............................gr. x.
Extracti Cinchona F..................................ℨiv.

Note—The potassium iodide forms potassio mercuric iodide with the bichloride of mercury. This is an alkaloidal precipitant and precipitates the alkaloids out of the fluid extract of cinchona.

22. Criticize this Prescription:

R Liquoris Plumbi Subacetatis...................fℨiv.
Mucilaginis Acaciae.............................fℨvi.
Aquae...... ....q. s. fℨvj.

Note.—The solution of lead subacetate precipitates the mucilage.

23. Criticize the following Prescription:

R Argenti Oxidi........................ ....gr. viij.
Creosoti ....gtts. xij.
Extracti Gentianae............................q. s.
M Fiat pilulae, No. xii.

Note.—Silver oxide will explode when mixed with organic substances. Use valaline as an excipient, and leave out the extract of gentian.

24. Complete the following Prescription.

R Hydrargyri Bichloridi ....q. s.
Aquae Destillata...................................fℨiv.
Misce. Fiat solutio (1-1000).

Note.—Dissolve 1.82 gr. of mercuric chloride in the required amount of water.

25. How much of the active ingredient should be used in the following?

℞ Cacainae Hydrochloratis..............................q. s.
Aquae Destillata.................................1000 c. c.
Misce. Fiat solutio (4%)

Note.—Use 40 grains of cacaine hydrochlorate.

26. How would you mix this?

℞ Sacchari...gr. lx.
Potassii Chloratis.............................gr. xx.
Acidi Tannici....................................gr. xl.
Fiat pulvis.

Note.—Mix on paper, with a bone spatula, to avoid an explosion.

27. What will the precipitate be in this Prescription?

℞ Potassii Iodidi..............................Ʒiiss.
Tincturae Ferri Chloridi ....f Ʒvi.
Syrupi ....f Ʒiv.
Aquae Destillata...........................f ℥iv.
Misce.
Signa.   Ut dictum.

Note.—There will be a black precipitate of free iodine. The mixture
is a dangerous combination and should never be dispensed.

28. Criticize this Prescription:

℞ Bismuthi Subnitratis.....................gr. xl.
Sodii Bicarbonatis..........................gr. xx.
M. Fiat pilulae, No. xx.

Note.—The bismuth salt it liable to have an acid reaction and by decomposing the sodium bicarbonate may cause the pills to explode.

29. How would you fill this Prescription?

℞ Acidi Salicylici ....3ij.
    Potassii Bicarbonatis.... ....gr. lx.
    Vini Colchici R.............................. ....f3iv.
    Aquae...ad. 3iv.

Note.—Potassium bicarbonate is decomposed by the salicylic acid.
Mix in an open vessel to allow the carbon dioxide to escape. Cork
the bottle loosely.

30. Criticize this Prescription:

℞ Quininae Sulphatis.........................gr. xxx.
    Acid. Sulph. Dil.......... :...........................q. s.
    F. E. Glycyrrhizae ....ad. 3ij.

Note.—The names of the ingredients should all be abbreviated or all
written in full. The fluid extract of glycyrrhiza was evidently
added to mask the taste of the quinine, but by using the acid to dissolve the quinine the sweet principle is precipitated and the preparation made more bitter.

Chemistry.

The elementary substances of interest to Pharmacy, with their symbols, valence and atomic weights.

	VAL.	AT. WT.	SYM.
Antimony	III.V.	120.	Sb.
Arsenic	III.V.	75.	As.
Barium	II.	137.9	Ba.
Bismuth	III.	209.	Bi.
Bromine	I.	80.	Br.
Calcium	II.	40.	Ca.
Carbon	IV.	12.	C.
Chlorine	I.	35.5	Cl.
Copper	I.II.	63.	Cu.
Gold	I.III.	196.5	Au.
Hydrogen	I.	1.	H.
Iodine	I.	127.	I.
Iron	II.VI.	56.	Fe.
Magnesium	II.	24.	Mg.
Mercury	I.II.	200.	Hg.
Oxygen	II.	16.	O.
Potassium	I.	39.	K.
Silver	I.	108.	Ag.
Sodium	I.	23.	Na.
Sulphur	II.	32.	S.
Zinc	II.	65.	Zn.

Acid Hydrochloric ....HCl

Acid Nitric ....HNO_3

Acid Sulphuric	H_2SO_4
Acid Sulphurous	H_2SO_3
Acid Nitrous	HNO_2
Acid Acetic	$HC_2H_3O_2$
Acid Boric	H_3BO_3
Acid Phosphoric	H_5PO_4
Alcohol	C_2H_5OH
Ammonia	NH_3
Glycerin	$C_3H_5(OH)_3$
Lime	CaO
Mercuric Chloride	$HgCl_2$
Mercurous Chloride	Hg_2Cl_2
Potassium Iodide	KI
Potassium Bromide	KBr
Potassium Bicarbonate	$KHCO_3$
Caustic Potash	KOH
Hydrocyanic Acid	HCN
Silver Nitrate	$AgNO_3$
Sodium Bicarbonate	$NaHCO_3$
Sodium Chloride	$NaCl$
Sugar	$C_{12}H_{22}O_{11}$
Water	H_2O
Carbon Dioxide	CO_2
Carbon Monoxide	CO
Citric Acid	$H_3C_6H_5O_7$
Benzoic Acid	$HC_7H_5O_2$
Salicylic Acid	$HC_7H_5O_3$
Calcium Hydrate	$Ca(OH)_2$
Calcium Carbonate	$CaCO_3$

Acid Sodium Sulphate..NaHSO₄

Ammonium Sulphate................................ ....(NH₄)₂SO₄

---

1. *What is Chemistry?

Chemistry is that science which treats of the elements found in nature, their properties, compounds, actions and reactions upon one another.

2. *What is an Element?

A substance that cannot by any known means be divided into two or more simpler substances.

3. *What is a Chemical Compound?

A chemical compound consists of two or more elements chemically combined in definite proportions.

4. *What is Matter?

Anything that occupies space, or has length, breadth or thickness.

5. *In how many forms does Matter exist?

Three: solid, liquid and gaseous.

6. Define a Solid?

A solid body is one in which the particles of matter are attracted so strongly that the body maintains its form under all ordinary circumstances.

7. What is a Liquid Body?

A liquid body is one in which the particles of matter are so feebly attracted together that they move upon each other with the greatest facility. Hence, a liquid can never be made to assume any particular form, except that of the vessel in which it is enclosed.

8. What is a Gas?

A body in which the repellent forces are greater than the attractive forces, consequently gases always tend to occupy a larger space.

9. *What is Chemism?

An attractive force which is exerted between the atoms causing them to unite.

10. *What is Cohesion?

Cohesion is that force which binds together molecules of the same kind to form one uniform mass.

11. *What is Adhesion?

Adhesion is that form of attraction which exists between unlike particles of matter when in contact with each other.

12. *What is the law of Definite Proportions?

Any given chemical compound always contains the same elements in the same proportion by weight.

13. *What is an Atom?

An atom is the smallest particle of matter that can enter into a chemical reaction.

14. *What is a Molecule?

A molecule is the smallest particle of matter that can exist in the free state.

15. *What is a Symbol?

A symbol is an abbreviation standing for the name of an element.

16. *What is a Formula?

A formula is a symbolic expression of the constituents of a molecule.

17. *What is Valence?

Valence is the degree of combining power of an atom as compared with hydrogen.

18. *What is understood by Combining Number or Atomic Weight?

It expresses the proportion by weight in which an element enters into combination.

19. How are Atomic Weights determined?

By the specific gravity of elements and compouuds in the form of gas or vapor.

20. In estimating the Weights of Elements, what one is taken as the standard?

Hydrogen.

21. Is Hydrogen a solid, liquid, or gas?

Gas.

22. *What elementary substance is essential to all animal life?

Oxygen.

23. What is Ozone?

An allotropic form of oxygen.

24. *How is Hydrogen prepared?

By acting on zinc with sulphuric acid, according to following equation:

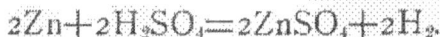

$$2Zn + 2H_2SO_4 = 2ZnSO_4 + 2H_2.$$

25. What important compound is formed by the combination of Hydrogen and Nitrogen?

Ammonia, NH_3.

26. What important article of commerce is made by dissolving NH_3 in water?

Aqua Ammonia.

27. *What is formed when Oxygen and Hydrogen combine chemically?

Water, H_2O.

28. What is produced when Hydrogen and Chlorine combine?

Hydrochloric Acid.

8h

29. *What is Oxidation?

The adding of oxygen to a substance.

30. *What is Reduction?

The taking away of oxygen from a body.

31. *What is Analysis?

Analysis is the resolving of a compound into its elements.

32. What is Synthesis?

Synthesis is the building up of a compound from its elements.

33. Name the two compounds of H and O ?

Water, Hydrogen Dioxide.

34. *What is Latent Heat?

Heat absorbed by a body before there is a rise in the temperature. The heat is supposed to be used in rearranging the molecules.

35. What impurities are liable to be in Drinking Water?

Organic impurities, chlorides, ammonia.

36. *What are Binary Compounds?

Compounds which consist of but two elements.

37. *What is an Acid?

A salt of hydrogen, or the combination of an acidulous radical with hydrogen.

38. *What is a Base?

A substance that has the power to neutralize an acid.

39. *What is a Salt?

A salt is the product of the action of an acid on a base.

40. *What is an Acid Salt?

An acid salt is one which is formed by replacing only a part of the hydrogen of an acid by a base.

41. *What is a Normal Salt?

A normal salt is one that is formed by replacing all of the hydrogen of an acid by a metal.

42. *What is a Basic Salt?

A normal salt of a metal combined with the oxide or hydrate of the same metal.

43. *What is an Alkali?

The stronger bases are known as alkalies. They have the power of neutralizing acids and of turning red litmus paper blue.

44. How are Temperature and Pressure of the Atmosphere measured?

(a) Temperature by the Thermometer.
(b) Pressure by the Barometer.

45. *What is the chief use of Nitrogen in the air?

To dilute the oxygen.

46. What impurities does the Air contain?

Carbon dioxide, ammonia, ozone, dust and smoke.

47. Name three forms of Free Carbon?

Diamond, graphite and coal.

48. What is Absolute Zero?

273 degrees below zero Centigrade. At this temperature all molecular motion ceases.

49. What is the rule for finding the weight of a liter of gas?

Multiply one-half the molecular weight by .0896.

50. *What effect has Temperature on the Volume of gas?

A rise of temperature increases the volume, a fall in temperature decreases the volume.

51. *Distinguish between Choke Damp and Fire Damp?

Choke damp is carbon dioxide. It is non-combustible. Fire damp is methane or marsh gas. When mixed with air it is highly explosive.

52. *What is Avogadro's Hypothesis?

Equal volumes of bodies in the form of gas or vapor under the same conditions contain an equal number of molecules.

53. Name the Halogens?

Bromine, Chlorine, Iodine and Fluorine.

54. Explain how Chlorine acts as a bleaching agent?

It only acts in the presence of water (H_2O); the chlorine combines with the hydrogen and liberates the oxygen, and while it is in the free state it readily combines with organic coloring matter and destroys it.

55. What is the Molecular Weight of a compound?

The sum of the weights of the atoms.

56. *What is produced when an Oxide salt is acted upon by an Acid?

The product is a salt of the metal and acid radical with a by-product of as many molecules of water as there are oxides present.

57. *What is produced by acting on a Carbonated salt with an Acid?

When a carbonated salt is acted upon by an acid the product is a salt of the metal and acid radical with a by-product of as many molecules of water and carbon dioxide as there are carbonates present.

58. *What is the result of acting on a Salt of an Organic acid with a strong Mineral acid?

The product is a salt of the metal and mineral acid, and the organic acid is set free.

59. *How would you join an acid radical with a metal?

Use the valence of one as the sub-figure of the other.

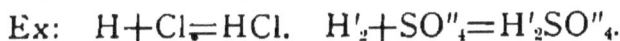

Ex: $H+Cl \rightleftharpoons HCl.$ $H'_2+SO''_4=H'_2SO''_4.$

60. What is the test for Nitrites?

(a) Nitrites bleach a solution of Potassium Permanganate.
(b) When acidulated with acetic acid they give a white precipitate with silver nitrate.

61. *What is the test for HCl and Chlorides?

Silver nitrate gives a white precipitate, insoluble in HNO_3 but soluble in ammonia.

62. *What is the test for Iodides?

Treat the iodide with chlorine water, add starch paste. The starch will be colored a deep blue.

63. Give the test for Carbonates.

Carbonates effervesce with all strong acids.

64. How is "H_2S," Hydrogen Sulphide, distinguished?

By its odor and by its blackening paper which has been moistened with a solution of lead acetate.

65. What is the test for Benzoates?

Neutral solutions give a flesh colored precipitate with test solution of ferric chloride.

66. What is the test for Salicylates?

They give a red solution with test solution of ferric chloride.

67. *Give the test for Citrates.

Citrates give a white precipitate with silver nitrate, which does not blacken on bo ling.

68. *What is the test for Tartrates?

Tartrates give a white precipitate with silver nitrate, which turns black on boiling. When tartaric acid is ignited it gives the odor of burnt sugar.

69. *How would you test for NH_3?

It is liberated by strong alkalies, like caustic soda, recognized by its odor.

70. What is the test for Sodium Salts?

The sodium salts color an alcohol flame intensely yellow.

71. *How would you distinguish Ferrous from Ferric Salts?

Potassium ferricyanide gives a blue color with ferrous salts, and an olive green color with ferric salts.

72. *Give a reliable test for Lead Salts.

H_2SO_4 gives a white precipitate with salts of lead. The precipitate is insoluble.

73. *How would you test for Salts of Mercury?

(a) Potassium Iodide gives a green precipitate with mercurous salts and a red precipitate with mercuric salts.

(b) A plate of copper placed in a solution of mercury will be coated with the metal.

74. *How would you test for Arsenic in the presence of Antimony?

Heat a strong solution of caustic soda in a test-tube. Add zinc and the solution containing the arsenic and antimony. Place over the mouth of the tube a piece of filter paper moistened with test solution of silver nitrate. If arsenic is present the spot of silver will be blackened.

75. *How would you determine the strength of Acids?

By volumetric alkali solution.

76. *How would you determine the strength of Alkalies?

By volumetric acid solution.

77. What is the official name of this formula? $Al_2K_2(SO_4)_4, 24H_2O$?

Alumen.

78. Name three salts of Zinc that are official.

Zinci Carbonas Praecipitatus, Zinci Acetas, Zinci Bromidum.

79. *In what Pharmacopoeal process is the Cyanide of Silver made use of?

In the extemporaneous preparation of hydrocyanic acid.

80. Give formulae for Calomel and Corrosive Sublimate.

Hg_2Cl_2, Calomel. $HgCl_2$, Corrosive Sublimate.

81. How is White Precipitate prepared?

By adding ammonia water to a solution of corrosive sublimate.

82. What soluble compound of Antimony is recognized in the U. S. P.?

Antimonii et Potassii Tartras.

83. How can Gases be liquified?

By pressure.

84. *Define Calorie.

It is the amount of heat necessary to raise the temperature of one gram of water one degree Centigrade.

85. What is Spontaneous Combustion?

When organic substances are oxidized with sufficient rapidity to raise the temperature to the point of ignition, the process of burning is known as spontaneous combustion.

86. What is an Oxide?

A binary compound of oxygen.

87. How is Glacial Acetic Acid made?

By distilling fused sodium acetate with concentrated sulphuric acid. The distillate is glacial acetic acid.

88. What advantage has $NaClO_3$ over $KClO_3$?

It is sixteen times more soluble.

89. How is Phosphoric Acid prepared?

By acting on phosphorus with bromine and dilute nitr'c acid.

90. What official compound contains Sulphur loosely combined?

Carbon Disulphide.

91. What are the functions of a Chemical Symbol?

(a) It is shorthand for the name of the element.
(b) It represents one atom of the element.
(c) It stands for a constant weight of the element.
(d) Symbols represent single and equal volumes of gaseous elements.

92. What are the functions of a Chemical Formula?

(a) It indicates the names of the elements.
(b) Its symbol or symbols, together with the sub-figures, show the number of atoms in the molecule.
(c) It stands for a constant weight of a compound, the molecular weight.
(d) It represents two volumes of the substance, if volatilizable, in the state of gas or vapor, and the number of volumes of gaseous elements from which two volumes of any gaseous compound were obtained.

93. How is Chemical Force distinguished from other forces?

Chemical force is exerted only between definite weights and volumes of matter, and it produces an entire change of properties in the bodies on which it is exerted.

94. Distinguish between Carbonates, Hydrocarbons and Carbohydrates.

(a) Carbonates are compounds that contain the group CO_3.
(b) Hydrocarbons are compounds of carbon and hydrogen.
(c) Carbohydrates are carbon compounds that contain hydrogen and oxygen in the proper proportion to form water.

95. Give three rules governing the formation of salts.

(a) The direct union of two elements forms salts that end in "*ide.*"

(b) Acids ending in "*ous*" unite with bases to form salts that end in "*ite.*"

(c) Acids that end in "*ic*" unite with bases to form salts that end in "*ate.*"

URINARY ANALYSIS.

96. What is the object of Analyzing Urine?

To detect the presence of abnormal constituents and to determine an excess or deficiency of the normal constituents.

97. What are the most common Abnormal constituents.

Albumen, blood, pus, bile and sugar.

98. What reaction has Urine?

Fresh urine has a slightly acid reaction.

99. Turbidity in fresh Urine may be due to what?

Turbidity may be due to urates, phosphates, or pus. Urates redissolve when the urine is warmed, phosphates redissolve on the addition of acetic acid; pus is detected by the microscope.

100 What should be the Specific Gravity of Urine?

From 1.015 to 1.025. Any considerable deviation from these limits would suggest a possible pathological condition.

101. How would you test for Albumen in Urine?

Place a small quantity of urine in a test-tube, add a drop of acetic acid and apply heat in such a manner that the upper portion only of the fluid will be heated. If albumen is present the urine will become turbid, more or less so in proportion to the amount of albumen present.

102. How would you test for Albumen by the use of Nitric Acid?

Place a small quantity of nitric acid in a test-tube, then pour the urine in in such a way that it will float upon and not mix with the acid. A white zone will form at the line of contact of the two liquids if albumen is present.

103. How would you test for Blood in Urine?

Urine containing blood is usually high colored and the corpuscles appear under the microscope as reddish circular discs, either single or laid together in strings resembling piles of coin. Blood may also be detected by adding tincture of guaiac and an aqueous solution of peroxide of hydrogen to the urine. If blood is present the mixture will turn blue; the rapidity of formation of which depends upon the amount of blood present.

104. How would you detect Pus in the Urine?

The presence of pus is easily detected by the microscope. Urine containing pus will effervesce with hydrogen peroxide.

105. Give two reliable tests for Sugar in Urine.

Add picric acid solution and liquor potassa to the urine and boil. If sugar is present a dark mahogany color will be developed.

To a portion of clear urine in a test tube add a few drops of solution of copper sulphate; add solution of potash or soda until the precipitate first formed is redissolved, then slowly heat the solution to near the boiling point. A yellowish-red or red precipitate will form if sugar is present.

106. What is the test for Bile in Urine?

Add sulphuric acid and sugar and apply heat. If bile is present the color will change from cherry red to purple, or give a play of colors.

Miscellaneous.

Questions on Pharmacy and Chemistry.

1. *What is Pharmacognosy?

Pharmacognosy is that branch of the study of medicines which treats of the natural origin, appearance, structure and other means of identification of organic drugs.

2. What is Therapetics?

The science of applying medicines.

3. What is Microscopy?

The study which treats of the microscope and its uses.

4. *What is a Menstruum?

The solvent used in the process of percolation is technically known by that name.

5. How may recovered distilled alcohol be purified?

By treating it with potassium permanganate, allowing it to stand for a few days and filtering.

6. What are the ingredients in Capsicum Plaster?

Oleoresin of Capsicum.
Resin Plaster.

7. *What is the formula for the official Suppository?

Glycerin.
Sodium Carbonate.
Stearic Acid.

8. What official preparations contain Vanilla?

Tincture of Vanilla.
Troches of Iron.

9. What is the official Triturate?

Trituration of Elaterin.

10. *What two proprietary preparations are official in the U. S. P?

Solol and Adeps Lanae Hydrosus.

11. *How are Aloes purified?

Heat the aloes on a water bath until melted; then mix them with alcohol, strain and evaporate until the mass becomes brittle when cooled.

12. *How is Turpentine deodorized?

By shaking the oil with lime water, then distilling the mixture, and separating the oil from the water.

13. *How is Resin of Guaiac prepared?

The resin is usually prepared by boiling guaiac chips in salt water, the resinous scum is collected, melted and strained.

14. *How is Croton Oil extracted from the seed?

By expression or by precolating the crushed seeds with carbon disulphide and distilling the percolate.

15. *In what different ways is Castor Oil extracted from the seed?

(a) By cold expression.
(b) By expression with heat.
(c) By percolation with alcohol.
(d) By decoction.

16. *How would you test for Nitrobenzol in Oil of Bitter Almond?

Treat the oil with potassium permanganate; if it is pure the odor will be destroyed, but if it contains Nitrobenzol it will still retain the odor of bitter almonds.

17. What is the test for Dementholized Oil of Peppermint?

The dementholized oil is nearly odorless and does not become thick and deposit crystals when subjected to a freezing temperature, difference from pure oil.

18. *How would you test for Cotton Seed Oil in Olive Oil or Lard Oil?

Shake a small quantity of the suspected oil in a test tube with an alcoholic solution of silver nitrate containing a few drops of nitric acid. If the oil is pure it should not become reddish or brown nor form a dark ring at the line of contact of the two liquids.

19. *What official preparation of Glycyrrhizin? How prepared?

Ammoniated Glycyrrhizin.
Prepared by extracting the glycyrrhizin with ammonia water. Pre-

cipitating it with sulphuric acid, washing and drying on plates of glass so that the finished salt may be obtained in scales.

20. What is the distinguishing test between powdered Acacia and powered Tragacanth?

Acacia is soluble in water, Tragacanth is only partially soluble.

21. *How is Carbon Disulphide purified?

By agitation with mercury and distillation in contact with white wax.

22. *Why is the oil boiled in the preparation of Phosphorated Oil; and why is Ether used?

(a) The oil is heated to expel air and traces of water, which would aid in oxidizing the phosphorus.

(b) The ether assists in the preservation of the preparation and renders the oil less disagreeable to the the taste.

23. How is "red" or Amorphous Phosphorus prepared?

It is prepared by allowing phosphorus to remain for several days in an atmosphere of carbon dioxide, at a temperature varying from 215° C. to 250° C.

24. *What is the chemical formula use and dose of Tri-iodomethane?

CHI_3. Used as an alterative, antiseptic and anaesthetic. Dose 3 gr.

25. *What is the test for Aldehyde in alcoholic liquids.

An alcoholic liquid that contains aldehyde will turn brown when mixed with potassium hydrate test solution.

26. What is the test for Tannin in Whiskey?

When more than traces of tannin are present it will turn dark green when treated with ferric chloride test solution.

27. *How would you test for acidity in Ether and Acetic Ether?

When they contain acid they will turn blue litmus paper red.

28. How would you clear a cloudy solution of Morphine Acetate?

Add Acetic Acid

29. What fat is miscible with water?

Hydrous Wool-Fat.

30. What is Magnesia of the U. S. P?

Magnesium Oxide.

31. *What is the chemical formula for Laughing Gas? How prepared?

N_2O. Prepared by heating ammonium nitrate and purifying the gas.

32. *What is Ethereal Oil?

A volatile liquid consisting of equal volumes of heavy oil of wine and ether.

33. How many Tinctures of Rhubarb are official? Give Latin name for each?

Three.
Tinctura Rhei.
Tinctura Rhei Dulcis.
Tinctura Rhei Aromatica.

34. What official salt is formed when a solution of Na_3CO_3 is added to a solution of $ZnSO_4$?

Zinci Carbonas Praecipitatus.

35. *What is Hall's Solution?

A solution of Strychnine, containing 1 gr. of Strychnine to the fluid ounce.

36. *What is Magendie's Solution.

A solution of Morphine containing 16 gr. of Morphine to the fluid ounce.

37. What official preparations contain Expressed Oil of Almond?

Phosphorated Oil.
Emulsion of Chloroform.
Ointment of Rose Water.

38. *How would you make Rochelle Salts?

Neutralize a solution of Potassium Bitartrate with Sodium Carbonate.

39. What are the official preparations of Jalap?

Extractum Jalapae.
Pulvis Jalapae Compositus.
Resina Jalapae.

40. What is the official preparation made from Opium?

Powdered Opium.

41. What are the official preparations of Capsicum?

Extractum Capsici Fluidum.
Oleoresina Capsici.
Tinctura Capsici.

42. *What three official salts of Salicylic Acid?

Sodium Salicylate.
Physostigmine Salicylate.
Lithium Salicylate.

43. *What is the difference between Calcium Chloride and Chloride of Lime?

(a) Calcium Chloride is a true salt of calcium, $CaCl_2$, made by acting on calcium carbonate with hydrochloric acid.
(b) Chloride of Lime is made by exposing calcium hydrate to the action of chlorine and has the chemical formula of $CaOCl_2$. The chlorine is very loosely combined.

44. *State the difference betwen Prepared Chalk and Precipitated Chalk.

(a) Prepared chalk is native friable calcium carbonate freed from its impurities by elutriation.
(b) Precipitated chalk is calcium carbonate made by precipitating a solution of calcium chloride with sodium carbonate.

45. What useful by-product is obtained when Myrrh is macerated with Alcohol?

The undissolved gum makes a good mucilage.

46. *Name two sources of Benzoic Acid.

(a) Found naturally in benzoin.
(b) Prepared artificially from the urine of cattle.

47. What is the distinguishing test between true Benzoic Acid and the Synthetic Acid.

The acid sublimed from benzoin has a lower melting point and is more soluble in water than the synthetic acid.

48. *What is the test for the purity of Castor Oil?

The oil should not acquire a blackish-brown color when shaken with a mixture of carbon disulphide and sulphuric acid.

49. What is Liquor Bismuthi?

An aqueous solution of bismuth made by dissolving bismuth and ammonium citrate in water with just enough of water of ammonia added to cause it to retain a faint odor of ammonia.

50. What official preparation is made direct from Sodium Carbonate?

Sodii Carbonas Exsiccatus.

51. *By what simple test can Dextrine be distinguished from Acacia?

By the odor. Dextrin has the odor of potato oil.

52. Why not use a high heat in the preparation of Oleate of Mercury?

A high heat would liberate metallic mercury.

53. *What is Auri et Sodii Chloridum? Use.

(a) A mixture of equal parts by weight of dry Gold Chloride and Sodium Chloride.
(b) Used as an alterative.

54. *What is Resorcin?   How prepared?

A diatomic phenol.

Usually prepared by fusing sodium benzol disulphonate with caustic
soda.

55. How is Salicylic Acid prepared commercially?

By treating sodium phenol with carbon dioxide.

56. *What is the difference between Scheel's HCy and
the U. S. P. HCy?

(a) Scheel's Acid contains about 5 per cent. of absolute HCy.
(b) The U. S. P. Acid contains 2 per cent. of absolute HCy.

57. *What menstruum is best to use in the preparations of Senna?   Why?

Water and diluted alcohol are the best solvents for the virtues of Senna. They extract the carthartic principles and leave the principles which cause griping. These would be extracted by strong alcohol and the cathartic principles would be left.

58. *What effect has heat on Rhubarb?

Heat changes its action from cathartic to astringent.

59. In what different forms is Ferrous Sulphate official?

Ferri Sulphas.
Ferri Sulphas Exsiccatus.
Ferri Sulphas Granulatus.

60. How is the Ferri Sulphas Granulatus prepared?

Granular ferrous sulphate may be made by adding a strong solution of
ferrous sulphate to alcohol, when it will be precipitated in the granular form.

61. What U. S. P. preparation is made by Elutriation?

Greta Praeparata.

62. *What are Elixirs?   What are the ingredients in
Aromatic Elixir?

9 i

Elixirs are aromatic, sweetened, spiritous preparations containing small quantities of active medicinal substances.

Aromatic Elixir contains:
Compound Spirit of·Orange.
Deodorized Alcohol.
Precipitated Calcium Phosphate.
Syrup.
Distilled Water.

63. *How many official liquors? In what different ways are they prepared?

(a) Twenty-four.
(b) Made by chemical solution in water and simple solution in water.

64. *By what two processes is Glycerine manufactured?

(a) As a by-product in the saponification of fats and oils in making soap or lead plaster.
(b) By decomposing fats and oils by pressure and superheated steam.

65. *How may Chloral be converted into Chloroform?

By treating an aqueous solution of it with a strong alkali.

66. *What effect has exposure on Spirits of Nitrous Ether? How can it be prevented?

When exposed it becomes acid. It may be kept neutral by adding a small quantity of sodium or potassium carbonate.

67. *What is the official name and the U. S. P. definition of Pyrogallic Acid?

(a) Pyrogallol.
(b) A triatomic phenol obtained chiefly by the dry distillation of gallic acid.

68. *What two official preparations contain Potassium Iodide in combination with Iodine? Why is it used?

Ointment of Potassium Iodide.
Liquor Iodi Compositus.
Used in both preparations to dissolve the iodine.

69. What are the U. S. P. Confections?

Confection of Rose.
Confection of Senna.

70. *What is Saponification?

The term is now extended in chemistry so as to include any process or reaction in which an alkali decomposes any ethereal salt or alkyl salt. (Atfield)

71. *What is the chemical difference between Sapo and Sapo Mollis?

Sapo is Sodium Oleate.
Sapo Mollis is Potassium Oleate.

72. What is the precipitate which forms in a solution of Lead Subacetate?

Lead carbonate caused by the absorption of carbon dioxide. It may be redissolved by adding acetic acid.

73. How can Tincture of Iodine be decolorized?

By adding sodium hyposulphite.

74. What effect does Nitric Acid have on Volatile Oils?

Strong nitric acid decomposes them.

75. What effect has Iodine on Volatile Oils?

The terpenes will explode with iodine.

76. *What is Amorphism?

A term used in chemistry to denote the absence of regular structure in a body.

77. *What are Isomeric Compounds?

Compounds consisting of the same elements in the same proportions, but having different properties.

78. Isomerism is of two kinds. Name them.

Metameric. Polymeric.

79. *Define each of the above terms.

(a) Metameric isomerism is a term applied to compounds which have the same percentage composition and the same molecular weights.

(b) Polymeric isomerism is a term applied to compounds which have the same percentage composition but different molecular weights.

80. *What is Isomorphism?

The quality of assuming the same crystalline form, though composed of different elements.

81. What is the chief source of Alcohol and how is it made?

(a) Corn and other grain containing starch.

(b) By mashing to convert the starch into sugar, fermenting to convert the sugar into alcohol and distillation to separate the alcoholic liquor. This liquor is the crude whisky from which alcohol is obtained.

82. What is the meaning of Assay?

To determine the amount of a given substance in a compound.

83. *What is meant by a Ferrous and Ferric Salt?

A Ferrous salt is one in which the iron exerts bivalent activity.
A Ferric salt is one in which the iron exerts trivalent activity.

84. What is a Sulphate?

It is a salt formed by the action of Sulphuric Acid on a base.

85. What is an Organic Acid?

An animal or vegetable acid.

86. What is Oleic Acid?

An organic acid obtained as a by-product in the manufacture of candles and glycerin.

87. What is a Mother Liquor?

The liquid remaining after crystals have formed.

88. *What is Aldehyde?

Aldehyde is alcohol from which two atoms of hydrogen have been extracted.

89. *How is Aldehyde made?

By acting on alcohol with oxidizing agents.

90. *How many Aldehydes can be produced?

Just as many aldehydes can be produced as there are alcohols to produce them from.

91. What acid would be formed by oxidizing Acetic Aldehyde?

Acetic Acid.

92. *What are the official derivatives of Aldehyde?

Paraldehydum, $C_6H_{12}O_3$.
Chloral, $C_2HCl_3O + H_2O$.
Chloroformum, $CHCl_3$.
Iodoformum, CHI_3.

93. *What is the chemical name for Chloroform?

Trichloro-methane.

94. *What is Chloral chemically?

Trichloraldehyde.

95. What is Iodoform chemically?

Tri-iodomethane.

96. What is the test for free Chlorine in Chloroform?

When chloroform is agitated with distilled water and the water separated it should not be affected by potassium iodide, T. S.

97. *What is the chief adulterant of Iodoform, with the test?

Picric acid is the chief adulterant. Detected by adding the iodoform to water. If picric acid is present the water will be colored yellow and the solution will also color silk or cotton cloth.

98. Write an equation for the manufacture of Ether?

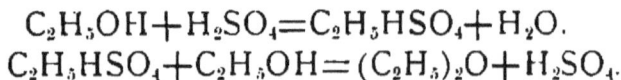

$$C_2H_5OH + H_2SO_4 = C_2H_5HSO_4 + H_2O.$$
$$C_2H_5HSO_4 + C_2H_5OH = (C_2H_5)_2O + H_2SO_4.$$

99. Write the chemical formula for Methyl Alcohol, Amyl Nitrite, Ethyl Nitrite?

(a) CH_3OH, (b) $C_5H_{11}NO_2$, (c) $C_2H_5NO_2$.

100. *What is an Alum?

When two trivalent and two univalent elements unite with a sulphate radical they always combine with twenty-four molecules of water and are called alums. As, $Al_2K_2(SO_4)_4.24H_2O$.

101. What is Iron Alum?

A form of alum in which the aluminum is displaced by iron. As, $Fe_2(NH_4)_2(SO_4)_4.24H_2O$.

102. *Why is HNO_3 used in the manufacture of Liquor Ferri Tersulphatis?

Used to change the iron from the ferrous to the ferric condition.

103. What is Quinine?

An alkaloid obtained from the bark of various species of Cinchona.

104. *What impurity is permitted in Quinine and how much?

The U. S. P. of 1890 allows it to contain a trace of the other Cinchona alkaloids. The U. S. P. of 1880 allowed one per cent.

105. *What are the official salts of Quinine?

Quinine Sulphate.
Quinine Bisulphate.
Quinine Hydrochlorate.
Quinine Hydrobromate.
Quinine Valerianate.

106. How is Quinine Bisulphate prepared?

Prepared by dissolving the quinine sulphate in dilute sulphuric acid, evaporating the solution and crystallizing the bisulphate.

107. *How would you prepare Hydrocyanic Acid extemporaneously?

By acting on silver cyanide with hydrochloric acid.

108. *What takes place when HCy is allowed to stand? What is the precipitate, and how can it be prevented?

When diluted hydrocyanic acid is kept in stock for a long time it becomes decomposed. A black precipitate is formed which contains paracyanogen. This decomposition may be prevented by the addition of a small quantity of sulphuric or hydrochloric acid.

109. How do you deodorize Iodoform?

By the use of coffee, tonka-bean or vanilla.

110. How would you test for Fusel Oil in Alcohol or Whiskey?

Add a small quantity to paper and evaporate; the last portion should not have a disagreeable odor.

111. *What are alcohols?

Alcohols are hydrates of hydrocarbon radicals.

112. *What are Ethers?

Ethers are oxides of hydrocarbon radicals.

113. *What are Compound Ethers?

They are salts formed by the action of acids on alcohols.

114. What are the chief adulterants of Arsenic?

Plaster of Paris and powdered glass.

115. What effect has exposure on salts made by calcination?

All salts made by calcination will absorb carbon dioxide and water from the air and go back into the hydrato carbonate.

116. How would you dissolve Starch?

Use a concentrated solution of zinc chloride or calcium chloride.

117. Why is Precipitated Zinc Carbonate made from hot solutions?

If cold solutions of zinc sulphate and sodium carbonate are mixed neutral zinc carbonate is formed. This carbonate quickly decomposes, carbon dioxide being evolved, which upon escaping makes a portion of the precipitate soluble. This loss is prevented by conducting the precipitate at the boiling point.

118. What menstruum is used in Syrup of Garlic?

Diluted Acetic Acid.

119. *What would you add to Cacao Butter for summer use?

Add wax to raise the melting point.

120. *What are Waxes?

They are fats of high melting points. Chemically they are compound ethers.

121. *What would you dispense for "Phenic Alcohol"?

Carbolic Acid.

122. *Why not dispense Sodium Hypophosphite with Salts of Silver or Mercury?

The sodium hypophosphite gives a white precipitate which would rapidly turn brown or black, owing to the liberation of the respective metals.

123. *What are Alkaloids?

Alkaloids are saline principles obtained from the animal and vegetable kingdoms. They are of definite chemical composition, alkaline reaction and possess the property of uniting with acids to form salts. They are generally the active constituents of the plants in which they are found.

124. *How are they divided with regard to their chemical composition?

Chemically they are either amides or amines.

125. *Which of the above classes are liquids and which solids?

The amides are solids.   The amines are liquids.

126. How do Alkaloids unite with Acids to form salts?

They unite as ammonia does, without displacing hydrogen; hence they are called compound ammonias.

127. *What is the test for Morphine?

Morphine turns red with nitric acid, and the acid is also colored.

128. *What is the test for Codeine?

When codeine is treated with nitric acid the crystals will turn red, but the acid even when warmed will only acquire a yellow color. Difference from and absence of morphine.

129. *What is the test for Strychnine?

Strychnine gives a play of colors when treated with potassium bi-chromate and sulphuric acid.

130. *How is Brucine detected in Strychnine?

When treated with nitric acid the acid should not turn more than faintly yellow (absence of brucine).

131. *What is the test for Quinine?

An aqueous acidulated solution of quinine when treated with bro-mine water and an excess of ammonia water will acquire an em-erald green color. In concentrated solutions it will form a green precipitate.

132. *How would you distinguish between Tannic Acid and Gallic Acid?

An aqueous solution of gallic acid should not precipitate alkaloids, gelatin nor albumen (difference from and absence of tannic acid).

133. What is the official Latin title of Ca and of CaO?

Ca is Calcium. CaO is Calx.

134. *What impurity is allowed in Potassium Bitartrate, and how much?

Calcium tartrate is permitted by the official test, if not in greater proportion than 1 per cent.

135. *What is Fermentation?

Fermentation is the process whereby new and useful compounds are formed by the decomposition of certain organic substances, when exposed to the action of water, air and a warm temperature.

136. *What is Putrefaction?

When offensive or worthless substances are formed by the decomposition of organic matter, it is called putrefaction.

137. *What causes Fermentation?

Authorities differ as to the cause. By some it is regarded as a chemical process. Others claim that it is due to the presence of very minute organisms.

138. *Into what two classes are Ferments divided?

(a) Organized, or physiological ferments.
(b) Unorganized, or soluble nitrogenous ferments.

139. What is produced when Sugar is allowed to ferment?

Alcohol and carbon dioxide.

140. How would you test for Alcohol in Oil of Lemon?

If the oil contains alcohol it will give a blue flame when burned in the dark.

141. What is Ether chemically?

Ethyl Oxide.

142. Syrup of Lime is an antidote to what three poisons?

Carbolic Acid, Creosote and Oxalic Acid.

143. *State why Animal Charcoal is sometimes objectionable as a Decolorizing agent?

When used to decolorize solutions containing organic matter it is liable to absorb the active constituents.

144. *What do you understand by Extractive?

Extractive is the peculiar principle of drugs that oxidizes and turns brown and almost always precipitates in liquid preparations.

145. How would you proceed to powder Nux Vomica?

First steam the drug, then dry it, after which it can be more readily powdered.

146. How should Terebenum be dispensed?

Either as an emulsion or in capsules.

147. *How should Cantharides be kept.

They should be kept in well-closed vessels and protected from mites by the addition of chloroform or carbon disulphide.

148. *How should Ergot be kept?

It should be only moderately dried, kept in a close vessel, and a few drops of chloroform added from time to time to prevent the development of insects.

149. How is Acetanilid prepared?

Acetanilid is made by heating a mixture of aniline and glacial acetic acid to the boiling point. The cooled congealed residue is purified by sublimation or recrystallization.

150. *What is the test between Carbolic Acid and Creosote?

Carbolic acid coagulates albumen or collodion. Creosote does not.

151 *What is the distinguishing test between a solution of Normal Lead Acetate and a solution of Lead Subacetate?

Normal lead acetate does not precipitate an aqueous solution of aca-

cia, but a solution of the subacetate forms a precipitate even in
very dilute solutions.

152. What infusions are made with cold water? By
what process are they made?

(a) Infusion of Cinchona.
    Infusion of Wild Cherry.
(b) Made by percolation.

153. *What are the Poisonous Liquors of the U. S. P.?

Liquor Acidi Arsenosi.
Liquor Arseni et Hydrargyri Iodidi.
Liquor Hydrargyri Nitratis.
Liquor Iodi Compositus.
Liquor Plumbi Subacetatis.
Liquor Potassi Arsenitis.
Liquor Sodii Arsenatis.
Liquor Zinci Chloridi.

154. What U. S. P. preparation contains Cochineal?

Compound Tincture of Cardamom.

155. Give two examples of upward precipitation.

Pepsin and Valerianate of Zinc.

156. How would you test for water in Alcohol?

Add anhydrous copper sulphate to the alcohol. If it contains water,
the copper sulphate will turn blue.

157. Give the Latin names of the two official Antidotes?

Ferri Oxidum Hydratum.
Ferri Oxidum Hydratum cum Magnesia.

158. What Salts of Morphine are official?

Morphine Acetate.
Morphine Sulphate.
Morphine Hydrochlorate.

159. Which is the most unstable salt of Morphine?

Morphine Acetate.

160. *Why is Nitric Acid used in Solution of Chloride of Zinc?

> Used to oxidize the iron so that it will be precipitated by the addition of the zinc carbonate.

161. What is formed by acting on Oil of Cloves with Potassium Hydrate?

> Potassium Eugenate, a substance closely allied to soap.

162. What official preparation is made by Circulatory Solution?

> Benzoinated Lard.

163. How would you prepare Benzoinated Lard for summer use?

> When Benzoinated Lard is to be kept or used during warm weather 5 per cent. or more of the lard should be replaced by white wax.

164. How many pints in a Liter?

> 2.11.

165. How many cubic centimeters in a Fluid Ounce?

> 30.

166. How should Pyroxylin be kept and why?

> Should be kept in paper boxes.
> When kept in air tight containers it undergoes spontaneous combustion.

167. How is the odor of Vanilla developed?

> By burying it in hot sand until it sweats.

168. What are Eclectic Resinoids?

> They are a class of preparations made by precipitating an alcoholic fluid extract of a drug by adding it to a large quantity of water and collecting the precipitate.

169. Are they the true active principles of the drugs?

They are not the true active principles although the names are often exactly the same. They vary greatly in strength and have been the cause of dangerous mistakes.

170. What causes the bleaching of the corks in bottles that contain Volatile Oils?

It is said by Remington to be due to ozone.
By Atfield to be due to Peroxide of Hydrogen.

171. What two acids in Opium?

Meconic Acid, Lactic Acid.

172. How is Glucose prepared artificially?

By acting on starch with very weak sulphuric acid.

173. How is H_2SO_3 made from H_2SO_4?

Heat sulphuric acid and charcoal together and pass the resulting sulphurous acid gas into distilled water.

174. What is the test between Alkaloids and Glucosides?

Glucosides in solution should not give a precipitate with tannic acid T. S. or other reagents for alkaloids. (Difference from and absence of alkaloids.)

175. What is Organic Chemistry?

The branch of chemistry that treats of the carbon compounds.

176. What is Apomorphine Hydrochlorate?

The hydrochlorate of an artificial alkaloid prepared from morphine or codeine.

177. What are Glucosides?

Glucosides are bodies mostly found in plants, which yield glucose as one of their products of decomposition when heated with a diluted mineral acid and water. They are sometimes the active principles of plants in which they are found, but they are more frequently combined resins, oils, alkaloids and bitter principles.

178. What is the test for Cane Sugar in Sugar of Milk?

Treat the sample of sugar with sulphuric acid, if it contains cane sugar it will turn black.

179. How are Granular Effervescent Salts made?

Granular effervescent salts are made by mixing the dry powders with dry tartaric acid and sodium bicarbonate and moistening the mixture with strong alcohol. The pasty mass is then passed through a sieve and the granules dried quickly in a hot room.

180. What are the principal adulterants of Sugar, with test?

(a) Prussian Blue and Ultramarine, used by refiners to save the expense of using bone-black.
(b) Neither an aqueous nor an alcoholic solution of sugar should deposit a sediment on prolonged standing.

181. What is Combustion?

Combustion is a variety of chemical combination in which the chemical union is sufficiently intense to produce heat and generally light.

182. What do you understand by Pulverization by Intervention?

Pulverization by intervention is the process of reducing substances to a powder, through the use of a foreign substance, from which the powder is subsequently freed by some simple method.

183. What is Caffeine Citrate?

It is simply a mixture of caffeine and citric acid.

184. What is the test for $HgCl_2$ in Hg_2Cl_2?

When Hg_2Cl_2 is washed with distilled water or alcohol the filtrate should not be affected by hydrogen sulphide T. S. or silver nitrate T. S. (absence of $HgCl_2$).

185. How is Oxalic Acid made?

By acting on cellulose, sugar or starch with nitric acid.

186. What action has Lead Oxide on Olive Oil?

When heated together they form a lead soap and glycerin.

187. Why is Charcoal used in the preparation of Potassium Iodide?

The charcoal is used to facilitate the deoxidation of the potassium iodate which is combined with the potassium iodide.

188. What effect has water upon Black Mustard?

When black mustard is treated with water the ferment, myrosin, becomes active and converts the potassium myronate into a pungent volatile oil which is, chemically, Allyl iso-thiocyanate.

189. What is Red Oil?

When red oil is ordered it may mean either crude oleic acid or crude oil of thyme.

190. How would you detect Potassium Iodate in Potassium Iodide?

Add some weak acid to the solution of potassium iodide, then add mucilage of starch; blue iodide of starch will be formed if potassium iodate is present.

191. How do Carbonates and Bicarbonates differ?

Bicarbonates contain double the amount of the group "CO_3" to a given amount of a base that carbonates do.

192. What is an Acidulous Radical?

A group of elementary substances which unite with hydrogen to form acids and with bases to form salts.

193. What are Oleates?

Oleates are liquid preparations made by dissolving metallic salts or alkaloids in oleic acid.

194. What are the numbers of the official Powders and what do they mean?

No. 20—Coarse.

No. 40—Moderately coarse.
No. 50—Moderately fine.
No. 60—Fine.
No. 80—Very Fine.

195. What is the difference between Dilute Alcohol in the U. S. P. of 1880 and the U. S. P. of 1890?

Dilute alcohol of 1880 was composed of equal parts by weight of alcohol and water; dilute alcohol of 1890 is equal parts by measure.

QUESTIONS WITHOUT ANSWERS.

196. Give a test for the identity of Chloral.

197. What is the difference between Sublimed, Washed and Precipitated Sulphur?

198. What is the difference in the properties of an Acid and an Alkali?

199. How would you distinguish chemically between Zinc Sulphate and Magnesium Sulphate?

200. Why does Chlorine not occur in the free state?

201. What is Dextro-glucose?

202. Outline a process for the preparation of Phosphorus Pills.

203. Give percentage composition of Potassium Bromide.

204. Name all the official preparation of Mercury.

205. Give percentage strength of all the official preparations that contain Metallic Mercury.

10 j

206. What do you understand by the term Solvent?

207. What is the chemical difference between Carbo Animalis and Carbo Ligni?

208. Prepare an outline of the Pharmacy Law in your State.

209. What is meant by the combining weight of an Element?

210. Distinguish between Permanent and Temporary hardness of water.

211. What Poisons does the Poison Law in your State require you to register?

212. Does the Poison Law of your State require you to keep a Poison Register?

213. What are Local Remedies?

214. What is the English name of this compound, $NH_4 HCO_3 NH_4 NH_2 CO_2$?

215. What is official Ammonium Carbonate, chemically?

216. How may Ammonium Bicarbonate be converted into Ammonium Carbonate?

217. What is the object of making a Syrup of Lime?

218. How is Syrup of Hypophosphites with Iron made?

219. What are the ingredients in Chalk Mixture?

220. Upon what does the activity of Chlorinated Lime depend?

221. How much water of crystallization does Magnesium Sulphate contain?

222. What is the formula for Magnesium Carbonate?

223. What variety of Sugar is found in Urine?

224. How would you detect Arsenic in Zinc?

225. How can Zinc Bromide be made?

226. How is Solution of Zinc Chloride freed from Iron?

227. What two rare metals are usually found in combination with Cerium?

228. In administering Magnesia, would you add the Magnesia to the diluent, water or milk, or the diluent to the Magnesia, and why?

229. What is the official name of this compound, $(MgCO_3)_4Mg(OH)_2$?

230. How is Bismuth Subnitrate prepared?

231. Give a brief description of Bismuth.

232. What are the ingredients in Wine of Antimony?

233. How would you antidote the above preparation?

234. What is Marsh's test for Arsenic?

235. How would you make Arsenous Acid?

236. What should be the per cent. of pure Acid in official Arsenous Acid?

237. Name some special forms of Cellulose.

238. What is No. 8 Acetic Acid?

239. What are some of the uses of Cellulose in Pharmacy?

240. How is the best Acetic Acid for medical purposes obtained?

241. What is the Latin official name of Tar?

242. How is Oil of Tar prepared?

243. What is "Salt of Sorrel" or "Essential Salt of Lemons?"

244. How do the above named salts act in removing iron rust from linen?

245. What color is produced when Iodine T. S. is added to Mucilage of Tragacanth?

246. What official preparation is made from Sassafras Pith?

247. What principle does Iceland Mass contain?

248. Under what name is Dextrin largely used in the arts?

249. How is Carmine prepared?

250. How can we distinguish between Glacial Acetic Acid and the weaker Acid?

251. What is the composition of Inulin?

252. What color reaction does it give with Iodine, and how does this differ from Starch?

253. What does Slippery Elm bark contain?

254. What sweet principle does Glycyrrhiza contain?

255. What sweet principle does Eriodictyon contain?

256. With what is Argenti Nitras Dilutus diluted?

257. What is the melting point of Petrolatum Spissum?

258. What three preparations contain free Chlorine, and what is the strength of each?

259. What four official preparations contain Tannic Acid?

260. What are the ingredients in Tincture of Ipecac and Opium?

261. What official preparation contains Morphine Sulphate?

262. What Acid is used in Lunar Caustic?

263. Would you use an Acetate in a solution that contained Quinine?

264. What official preparation is made from Barium Dioxide?

265. What official Salt is formed by acting on a solution of Corrosive Sublimate with KOH?

266. What is the best solvent for Sulphur?

267. What official preparations are made direct from Iron?

268. State the difference between Benzol, Benzene, Benzin and Benzoin.

269. What is the strongest Alcohol that can be made by fractional distillation?

270. What takes place when Tincture of Catechu is kept on hand, and how can it be prevented?

271. What do you understand by the maximum density of a liquid?

272. What official drug owes its activity to adhering impurities?

273. How many official Pills contain Aloes?

274. What is used in preparing Potassa with Lime?

275. How is Moist Ferric Hydrate prepared?

276. What are the ingredients in Aromatic Spirits of Ammonia?

277. What official preparation is made from Lemon Juice?

278. What is the per cent. of $AgNO_3$ in Argenti Nitras Dilutus?

279. What official preparation contains Dilute Hypophosphorous Acid? Why is it used?

280. What official preparations are made from Alum?

281. What three preparations contain MgO?

282. What are the official preparations of Phosphorus?

283. Give three reliable tests for the salts of Iron.

284. What U. S. P. preparation contains Quinine Sulphate.

285. What is Daturine?

286. What is a Filter?

287. What is Lixiviation?

288. What is Lotion or Displacement washing?

289. What is Repercolation?

290. What wine is made from a Fluid Extract?

291. Describe NH_4.

292. How do Copper and Silver occur in nature?

293. What is the official Salt of Copper?

294. Name the alcoholic preparations of Rhubarb.

295. What is Glycerin, chemically?

296. Name two vegetable and two metallic Emetics?

297. Give two sources of Acetic Acid.

298. What is the difference between Potassa and Potassium?

299. What is the difference between Alumen and Aluminum?

300. What is Barley Sugar?

301. What is the test for Methyl Alcohol in Ethyl Alcohol?

302. What is Bleaching Powder, chemically?

303. What four official preparations contain Castor Oil?

304. Name some U. S. P. drugs made by Sublimation?

305. What advantage has Ammonia over the fixed alkalies?

306. What is the use and dose of Sodium Phosphate?

307. What is the official salt of Cerium?

308. What are the U. S. P. requirements of Brandy?

309. Define destructive distillation and name two U. S. P. drugs made by the process.

310. How would you make an Emulsion of Croton Oil?

311. What is the test for Creosote?

312. Why can Syrup of Lime be made stronger than Lime Water?

313. What do you understand by Detannated Cinchona?

314. Name three official preparations made by Exsiccation.

315. What should be the strength of Infusions and Decoctions when not otherwise directed?

316. What is Milk of Lime?

317. What are Suppositories?

318. What is the objection to using Ointment of Chrysarobin?

319. What is an Anhydrous Salt?

320. How do cells increase in number?

321. What is an Impalpable Powder?

322. What Salt is formed when the fumes of Hydrochloric Acid come in contact with the vapors of Ammonia?

323. What is Gum Arabic, chemically?

324. What do you understand by the term Bumping?

325. What are the U. S. P. requirements of Jalap?

326. For what purpose are the Barium Salts used?

327. How many Alkaloids are found in Opium?

328. What is Milk of Asafoetida?

329. What is Hydrosulphuric Acid?

330. What Salt of Arsenic in Fowler's Solution?

331. What is Lac Sulphur?

332. How is Acetic Ether made?

333. What effect has Mercury on Gold?

334. What is an Amalagam?

335. What is Absolute Alcohol?

336. What is meant by the nascent state of an element?

337. What are Abstracts?

338. How many Alkaloids have been found in Cinchona Barks?

339. What Acids are found in Cinchona Barks?

340. What are the adulterants of Oil of Rose?

341. What are the official preparations of Purified Aloes?

342. What is Aloinum?

343. For what purpose was Stearic Acid made official?

344. Name several substances that are more soluble in cold water than in hot?

345. How would you decolorize Whiskey?

346. How can Tonka Bean be detected when used as an adulterant for Vanilla?

347. How would you test for Glucose in Honey?

348. For what purpose is Honey used in the Iron preparations?

349. What is Malic Acid?

350. What is formed when Nitric Acid comes in contact with the skin?

351. What do Sulphites change to when exposed to the air?

352. What is the true chemical name of Sodium Hyposulphite?

353. What general synonym has been given to the preparations of the Subacetate of Lead?

354. How was the first Glycerine obtained?

355. How is Ammonium Carbonate made?

356. How should all salts of Silver be kept, and why?

357. How would you antidote Silver Cyanide and how all other salts of Silver?

358. Why should Glucosides not be prescribed with free acids or emulsin?

359. What precaution should be taken in dispensing an aqueous solution of Carbolic Acid?

360. What is the source of Succinic Acid?

361. What is the Kinetic Theory?

362. How many atoms to the molecule in Arsenic and Phosphorus.

363. What are oxidizing agents?

364. How should Amyl Nitrite be dispensed?

365. Why is Chloral incompatible with alkalies?

366. How would you powder Cardamom Seed and why?

367. Why does a mixture of White and Black Mustard yield a more pungent volatile oil than either one does alone?

368. What principles in Coffee are destroyed by roasting?

369. For what purpose was Elastica made official?

370. Why is Glycerin used to adulterate Saffron?

371. What official oil can be used as a substitute for Olive Oil?

372. Why should Taraxicum be gathered in the autumn?

373. How is Soap mottled?

374. What is the curd on hard water when soap is used in it?

375. What is the objection to the use of Vaseline as a base for ointments?

376. Name several commercial varieties of Opium?

377. How does Apomorphine differ from Morphine?

378. What is the source of Cod Liver Oil?

379. Define Specific Volume?

380. What is the Latent Heat of water?

381. What is the Latent Heat of steam?

382. What is the composition and properties of Cyan-ogen?

383. Why is Atropia used as an antidote to Opium poisoning.

384. Name several varieties of the metal Iron?

385. What is Musk?

386. Define Chemical Decomposition?

387. What is Pepsin and what are the U. S. P. require-ments?

388. How many ounces in one Liter?

389. What is the composition of Donovan's Solution?

390. What is the source of Hydrous Wool-Fat?

391. Under the influence of water what will some oils deposit?

392. Define Theoretical Pharmacy and show in what respect is differs from Practical Pharmacy?

393. Complete the following chemical equations:
$$Ag+HNO_3=$$
$$KOH+I=$$

394. Give mode of preparation of Chloroform and of Ether.

395. What precaution is necessary in mixing Turpen-tine and Sulphuric Acid?

396. What is the result when Camphor and Chloral are rubbed together?
397. How is Methyl Alcohol manufactured?
398. How is Calomel prepared and purified?
399. How would you distinguish between Antimony and Arsenic?
400. How would you distinguish between Bromides and Chlorides?
401. Name five Alkaloidal precipitants.
402. Why is Vinegar of Opium less nauseating than the Tincture of Opium?
403. Iodoform should contain what percentage of Iodine?
404. Explain why Hydrochloric Acid is used in Lunar Caustic.
405. Give the U. S. P. definition of Adeps.

ERRATA.

Answer to question 39, page 8, should be "—40°F."

Section "(a)", in answer to question 272, page 34, should be, "Arabin, a soluble gum found in Acacia."

Contents.

CONTENTS.

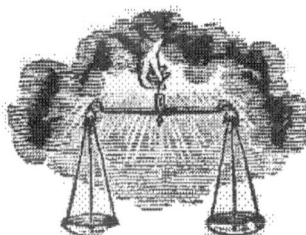